This Book Will Put You to Sleep

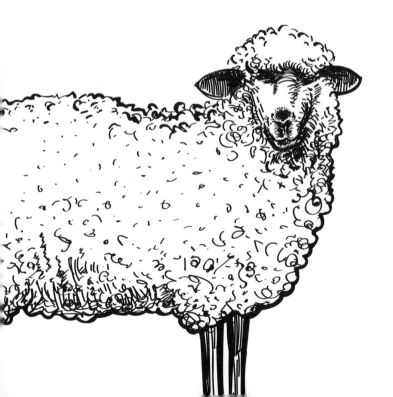

This Book

✦ Will ✦

Put You

to Sleep

Professor K. McCoy *&* Dr Hardwick

CHRONICLE BOOKS
SAN FRANCISCO

First published in the United States in 2018 by Chronicle Books LLC.

First published in the United Kingdom in 2018 by Ebury Press, a division of the Penguin Random House Group. Copyright © 2018 by Professor K. McCoy and Dr Hardwick. All Rights Reserved. No part of this book may be reproduced in any form without written permission form the publisher.

Library of Congress Cataloging-in-Publication Data

Names: McCoy, K., author. | Hardwick, Dr., author.

Title: This book will put you to sleep / Professor K. McCoy & Dr Hardwick.

Other titles: This book will send you to sleep

Description: San Francisco, CA : Chronicle Books, 2018. | First published in the United Kingdom in 2018 by Ebury Press, a division of the Penguin Random House Group. Copyright (c) 2018 by Professor K. McCoy and Dr Hardwick under the title "This book will send you to sleep."

Identifiers: LCCN 2018043268 | ISBN 9781452173610 (hardcover : alk. paper)

Subjects: LCSH: English wit and humor.

Classification: LCC PN6175 .M43 2018 | DDC 828/.9202—dc23 LC record available at https://lccn.loc.gov/2018043268

Manufactured in China

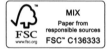

Illustrations on pages 12, 20-21, 28-29, 36, 58-59, 68-69, 96-97 by Diane Law Illustration on cover (and throughout) serg_65/Shutterstock.com; background image on cover BrankaVV/Shutterstock.com; page 11 Bodor Tivadar/Shutterstock.com; page 23 SAHAS2015/Shutterstock.com; page 38-39 vectorplus/Shutterstock.com; page 62-63 Vorobiov Oleksii 8/Shutterstock.com; page 91 Niagara705/Shutterstock.com; page 103 corbac40/Shutterstock.com; page 133 Babich Alexander/Shutterstock.com; page 175 Danussa/Shutterstock.com

Cover design and typesetting by Neil Egan

10 9 8 7 6 5 4 3

Chronicle Books LLC
680 Second Street
San Francisco, CA 94107
www.chroniclebooks.com

Chronicle Books publishes distinctive books and gifts. From award-winning children's titles, bestselling cookbooks, and eclectic pop culture to acclaimed works of art and design, stationery, and journals, we craft publishing that's instantly recognizable for its spirit and creativity. Enjoy our publishing and become part of our community at www.chroniclebooks.com.

Contents

Introduction

In our many years of research at the Institute of Pointless Studies, one important question that we have tried to address is the problem of insomnia and insufficient sleep. If you are trying to get sufficient sleep, it is important to have as little mental stimulation as possible. The most desirable state of mind to cultivate is one of boredom, lassitude and disinterest. As part of our research we have studied hypnotic states, somnambulism, stereotypical lethargy, mind-decelerating pharmacology and devoid phenomenology. In one five-year experiment, Professor K. McCoy encouraged her subjects to spend 15 hours a day in a darkened room listening to white noise and meditating on the void. Unfortunately none of the subjects were willing to continue to the end of the experiment, but the preliminary results in terms of sleep were most encouraging.

While some of the traditional methods of getting to sleep, such as counting sheep or listening to sounds of ocean waves, have had erratic results in experimental settings, we have established that the most consistently successful strategy is to read a book until you achieve a state of sufficient sleepiness. The challenge is to avoid books that are too exciting or intriguing, as the last thing you want when you are preparing for sleep is powerful mental stimulation. Many novels or works of nonfiction have at least some ability to fascinate the reader and to provoke unwanted trains of thought which, if not checked, may spiral into a state of dreadful wakefulness.

As a response to this discovery we compiled this collection of short texts. Each page is guaranteed to be devoid of excitement. All challenging or stimulating elements have been removed, and we have endeavoured to set and design the text in such a way as to befuddle the mind, inducing a state of hypnotic dreaminess and languor. The text has been prepared by a team of high-grade bores, emotionless drones and experts in dispiritingly pointless areas of academia. Professor McCoy's illustrations and designs add an additional layer of soporific confusion which is guaranteed to induce a powerful state of lethargy. In experiments, these texts have put 97 per cent of subjects to sleep within ten minutes 58 per cent of the time in 73 per cent of the conditions studied within an acceptable range of experimental error. Consequently we have gathered these experimental texts together into this book. We sincerely hope you find it as boring to read as we did to write it.

Professor K. McCoy and Dr Hardwick

The Political Crisis in Belgium, 2007–2011

The 2007–11 political crisis was a period of instability in Belgium. The issues that provoked the crisis included the question of state reform, and whether the electoral district Brussels-Halle-Vilvoorde should remain as a single electoral district, or be separated into two electoral districts. Following the 2007 elections there were 196 days of negotiations before a coalition could be formed. However, after the 2010 elections, there was an even longer period of 541 days' negotiation before a coalition could be formed. During these negotiations, a wide variety of Belgian politicians took charge of the discussions, in a variety of political roles. Bart De Wever of the New Flemish Alliance was in charge of the talks from 17 June 2010 to 8 July 2010 in the role of *informateur*. The title of *formateur* is used in Belgium to refer to the person who steers negotiations about a coalition government. The job of an *informateur* is to conduct preliminary talks that will lay the groundwork for the subsequent work of a *formateur*.

After De Wever, Elio Di Rupo of the Socialist Party became *pre-formateur*, a title that also refers to someone who lays the groundwork for a *formateur*, but who is not identified as *informateur* since he may go on to become *formateur* or even prime minister himself (while *informateurs* are more properly regarded as actual or potential assistants to the *formateur*). Di Rupo was in charge of the talks until 3 September 2010, after which he was replaced by Danny Pieters and André Flahaut who were Presidents of the Senate and the Chamber of Representatives respectively. They were jointly referred to as *mediators*, rather than as *formateurs*, *informateurs* or *pre-formateurs*. When their talks collapsed on 5 October 2010, De Wever took charge of the talks once more, but now instead of being known as the *informateur*, he was the *clarificator*. From 21 October 2010 to 26 January 2011 Johan Vande Lanotte became mediator and the talks continued.

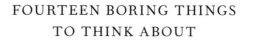

FOURTEEN BORING THINGS
TO THINK ABOUT

Watching 10 square feet (.93 square meter) of paint dry

Watching 12 square feet (1.11 square meters) of grass grow

A best practices city council rules-of-order conference seminar

Soil sample differentiation

The lunchtime line at a short-staffed post office

Office database training day

Snail races

Standard Income Deduction Form 52-A part 7

Fifty shades of beige

A sunday afternoon in 1975

The evaporation of 1 pint (.47 liter) of water in real time

The hum of electricity pylons

The longest game of Monopoly in human history

Confirming by counting the thread count of your sheets

The Administrative Bureaucracy of the Byzantine Empire

(An extract from *Byzantium: the Complete Administrative Guide* by Prof. L. Tedioso)

The civil service of the Byzantine Empire was a part of the Byzantine political culture but also separate from it. It had an administrative function, but also an executive approach to administration. The bureaucracy was reorganised many times over the years, as we shall see in much more detail on p.17, p.84, p.835, p.739 and p.1008. The civil service can be categorised in three sections: the palatine administration, based at a palace; the provincial government, which was responsible for government in the provinces; and the central civil service, which was responsible for central direction of the administrative bureaucracy. The civil service has been estimated to have been staffed by at least 600 civil servants, across 13 different bureaux or departments of state. The fundamental categorisation within civil administrative bureaucracy was between Kritai, or judicial officers, and Sekretikoi, or financial officers. The Sekretikoi were overseen by a general controller known as the Sakellarios. The Sakellarios in turn were overseen by departmental overseers known as Logothetēs. The Logothetēs tou Genikou, for example, was a finance minister in charge of financial administrative bureaucracy, who was the overseer for the Sakellarios of the financial bureau who in turn were the overseers for the Kritai of the financial bureau within the civil administrative bureaucracy. Similarly the Logothetēs tou Dromou supervised the post office. The Kritai who worked on matters relating to the post office, and other matters of similar import, reported to the Sekretikoi of the post office section of the civil service. And the Sekretikoi in turn reported to the Logothetē tou Dromou.

Spot the Difference

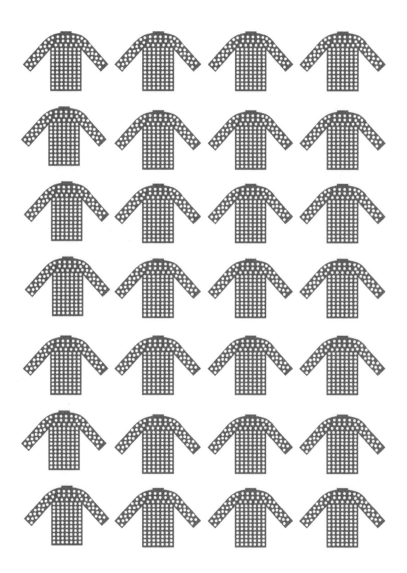

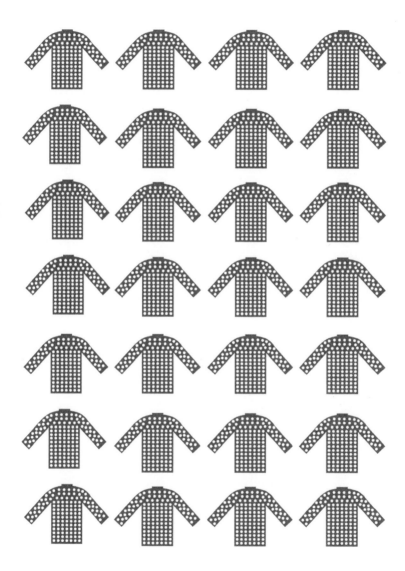

Multi-Storey Hypnosis

Close your eyes. You are walking along a concrete path, to the left of you is a concrete wall, to the right of you is a concrete wall. Right next to you on your left is a small blue car, next to it is a large grey car then a white car followed by a red car next to a green car with a bicycle in the back. Next to that is a silver car then a large black car with shiny wheels. Look to your right, there is a big grey car next to a medium-sized blue car next to a red car next to a large white van. Keep walking along the concrete path being mindful of the concrete walls on either side. As you walk you get to a concrete slope, go down the concrete slope, it's grey, very, very grey and it winds down and down. You are again on a concrete path, to the left of you is a concrete wall, to the right of you is a concrete wall. Directly to your left there is a red car next to a white car next to a large silver car with stickers on the windscreen. There are three black cars in a row followed by a green car then a tiny red car. To your left is a white car followed by a red van next to a small silver car with a baby seat in the back. Next is a yellow car followed by two silver cars and a large black motorbike. Keep walking along the concrete path. You get to another slope. Go down the slope, mindful of the grey walls on either side of you. Keep walking down and down as it goes round and round. You come to a concrete path. To the left of you is a concrete wall, to the right of you is a concrete wall. Directly next to you is a black car with a rack on the roof followed by a large blue van with blacked-out windows. Next to that is a white car followed by a green car followed by four silver cars. The first silver car is very small, the second silver car is large and shiny, and the third is medium-sized and hasn't been cleaned for a while, the fourth is small and has a cushion on the front seat. There is a large blue car followed by a white car and a small black van. Follow the path as it winds down and down …

40 NAMES FOR SNOW

Barchan

Blizzard

Corn

Cornice

Column

Crust

Dendrite

Finger drift

Firn

Flurry

Graupel

Ground blizzard

Grue

Hoarfrost

Lake-effect snow

Needle

New snow

Old snow

Onding

Penitents

Perennial snow

Pillow drift

Polycrystal

Powder

Rimed snow

Ripples

Roller

Sastrugi

Skift

Sleet

Slush

Snirt

Snow bridge

Snow drift

Snow squall

Snowburst

Snowflake

Snowpack

Snowstorm

Snowy snow

Some Sports Statistics

- In the 1886 World Series between the St Louis Browns and the Chicago White Stockings there was a total of 63 errors.

- The longest tennis match in history was between John Isner and Nicolas Mahut at Wimbledon in 2010. It lasted 11 hours and 5 minutes and was spread over the course of three days.

- In the 1958 World Men's Handball Championships Norway scored 67 goals.

- In the Archery category at the 1996 Olympics South Korea won one medal.

- In the world of cricket, the longest test match was played between South Africa and England, starting on 3 March 1939. It ended 12 days later, after 43 hours and 16 minutes of play, 1,981 runs and 5,447 balls. The result was a draw.

- In the Women's World Floorball Championships, Sweden has been crowned champion more than any other team. The only other winners have been Finland and Switzerland.

- In West Flanders and surrounding regions, a variant on the game of bowls is played. It is called tra-bowls.

- The World Championship for Rock Paper Scissors has a first prize of $10,000.

- In 2011, in the Northern Territory of Australia, the Staring Competition was won by Fergal 'Eyesore' Fleming, after 40 minutes and 59 seconds of staring without blinking at his opponent.

- One of the longest poker games ever was held at the Bird Cage Theatre in Tombstone, Arizona, from 1881 to 1889. It lasted 8 years, 5 months and 3 days.

- At the British and World Marbles Championship, glass marbles were first used instead of the previous clay marbles in April 1962.

- At the 1956 Olympics, in the Individual Dressage event, which was held in Sweden rather than Melbourne due to quarantine issues, the bronze medal was won by Liselott Linsenhoff of West Germany, riding Adular.

Mind Whirls: You Are Very Sleepy

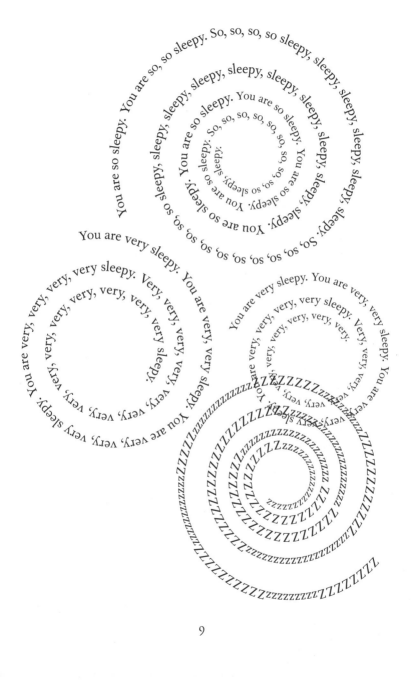

Recent Developments in the Taxonomy of Molluscs

Since the publication of the taxonomy of the Gastropoda by Bouchet & Rocroi (2005) there have been numerous minor developments in the way that scientists classify slugs and snails. One significant contribution made by Klussmann-Kolb and her colleagues was the reclassification of the Euthyneura. After further work by Jörger and colleagues, the major groups within the Heterobranchia were redefined. Obviously one of the most exciting new bits of research has been within the classification of the Conoidea, but we will return to this later.

It has recently been shown that the extinct taxon Helcionelloida is not a true gastropod, so these Paleozoic molluscs of uncertain position have been reclassified as a separate class within the Mollusca, to avoid confusion. Within the true limpet family (the Patellogastropoda), research by Nakano and Ozawa in 2007 has led to some minor reclassifications. The Acmaeidae have been absorbed into the identical Lottioidea but a new family, the Eoacmaeidae, has been defined. To increase the level of precision in this area of the taxonomy of the molluscs, three other families (Daminilidae, Lepetopsidae, Neolepetopsidae) are now part of the class Lottioidea.

When it comes to Vetigastropoda the 2009 work of Geiger has been significant. The subfamily Depressizoninae has been renamed as the family Depressizonidae. Two other groups previously regarded as subfamilies (the Larocheinae from the family Scissurellidae, and the Temnocinclinae from the family Sutilizonidae) have also been reclassified as families, but of course this involves an important piece of renaming. The Larocheinae are now known as the Larocheidae and the Temnocinclinae have been renamed Temnocinclidae.

One big piece of news is that while we used to believe that the superfamily Neomphaloidea was part of the clade Vetigastropoda, new developments in molecular phylogeny have shown that it actually belongs in its own clade, Neomphalina. However when it comes to the all-important relationship between Neomphalina and Vetigastropoda there is work remaining to be done, since the research is inconclusive.

Next, of course, we come to the Neritimorpha. In 2007, Bandel identified a number of new families within the Neritopsoidea, which he classified as part of the order Neritoina, which is itself in the superorder Cycloneritimorpha (but, naturally, still within the subclass Neritimorpha). This logically leads on to the recognition of Natisopsinae (identified as part of Neritopsidae by Bouchet & Rocrois in 2005) as part of the family Naticopsidae. So the superfamily Neritopsoidea now contains the families Neritopsidae, Fedaiellidae, Delphinulopsidae, Cortinellidae, Palaeonaricidae and Naticopsidae. On subsequent pages we will be discussing the importance of the taxonomy of Caenogastropoda and the revised relationship between the family Provannidae and the superfamily Abyssochrysoidea. We will also consider the elevation of the subfamily Semisulcospirinae to the more important status of family (for which it was renamed) Semisulcospiridae. Important as all of these developments with the taxonomy of molluscs are, it is worth bearing in mind that all classifications are subject to potential future reclassification.

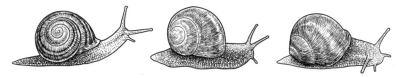

Sixteen Years of Growth Pattern in Holly (*Ilex aquifolium*)

YEAR 1

YEAR 2

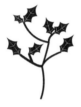

YEAR 5

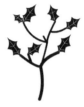

YEAR 6

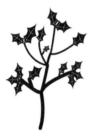

YEAR 9

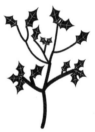

YEAR 10

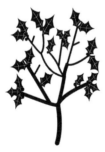

YEAR 13

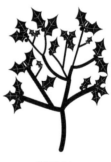

YEAR 14

YEAR 3

YEAR 4

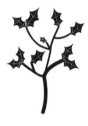

YEAR 7

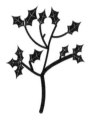

YEAR 8

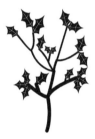

YEAR 11

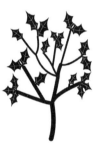

YEAR 12

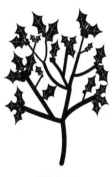

YEAR 15

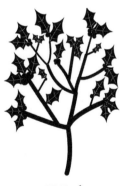

YEAR 16

Railway Gauges:
an Overview

Since the invention of steam trains in the nineteenth century, tracks have been built in various different sizes of gauge. (Gauge is a measure of the distance between the tracks.) George Stephenson built the Stockton and Darlington Railway with a gauge of 4 foot 8 inches, having used the same gauge for testing on the Killingworth Wagonway. This in turn was based on a mine tramway called the Willington Way.

Different gauges were used for different railways in the United Kingdom at the time. The Penydarren Tramroad in South Wales used a gauge of 4 foot 4 inches. The Monkland and Kirkintilloch Railway in Scotland used 4 foot 6 inches. The Dundee and Newtyle Railway, elsewhere in Scotland, used a gauge of 4 foot 6 and a half inches. The Redruth and Chasewater Railway used 4 foot. The Arbroath and Forfar Railway used a gauge of 5 foot 6 inches. The Ulster Railway used 6 foot 2 inches. However, following the opening of the Stockton and Darlington Railway many railways, including the Liverpool and Manchester Railway, used the same gauge as it had used, or in fact a very slightly larger one, 4 foot 8 and a half inches, which became known as standard gauge. It was also known as narrow gauge, in contrast to broad gauge, which was used by the Great Western Railway (7 foot initially, although this later changed to 7 foot and a quarter of an inch). There was some dispute as to whether narrow or broad gauge was better, while some railways continued to use other alternatives, for instance the Eastern Counties Railway used a gauge of 5 feet.

As railways spread around the world, a variety of gauges continued to be used. Some of the most common gauges were 3 foot 6 inches (used, for instance, in Southern and Central Africa, the Philippines, Japan and part of Australia), Russian gauge (4 foot 11 and $^{27}/_{32}$ inches – used in Armenia, Azerbaijan, Belarus, Estonia,

Finland, Georgia, Kazakhstan, Kyrgyzstan, Latvia, Lithuania, Moldova, Mongolia, Russia, Tajikistan, Turkmenistan, Ukraine and Uzbekistan), Finnish gauge (5 foot – used in Finland), Irish gauge (5 foot 3 inches – used in Ireland, Brazil and parts of Australia), Iberian gauge (5 foot 5 and $2\frac{1}{32}$ inches – used in Spain and Portugal) and Indian gauge (5 foot 6 inches – used in India, Pakistan, Bangladesh, Sri Lanka, Argentina and parts of the United States). Standard gauge was used in Albania, Argentina, Australia, Austria, Belgium, Bosnia and Herzegovina, Bulgaria, Canada, China, Croatia, Cuba, Czech Republic, Denmark, Djibouti, Ethiopia, France, Germany, Greece, Hungary, Indonesia, Israel, Italy, Liechtenstein, Luxembourg, Macedonia, Mexico, Montenegro, Netherlands, North Korea, Norway, Panama, Peru, Poland, Romania, Serbia, Slovakia, Slovenia, South Korea, Spain, Sweden, Switzerland, United States, Uruguay, Venezuela, and some lines in India, Japan and Taiwan.

Within the United States there was also some variation in the gauge used for railways. The standard gauge of 4 feet 8 and a half inches was widely used, for instance, on the Baltimore and Ohio Railroad and the Boston & Albany. The Pennsylvania Railway used a slightly different gauge of 4 feet 9 inches. The Erie Lackawanna used a broader gauge of 6 feet. Canadian railways used a gauge of 5 feet 6 inches. In the Southern states of the United States the most common gauge was 5 feet 0 inches. The transcontinental railroad was initially planned at 5 feet 0 inches but later on they changed the plan and used standard gauge, 4 feet 8 and a half inches.

Some interesting alternative gauge sizes that are no longer in use include 6 foot 4 and $\frac{5}{8}$ inches, used in the Netherlands between 1839 and 1864, 5 foot 9 and a quarter inch, used briefly in Indonesia, 4 foot 11 and $\frac{3}{8}$ inches, used in Ukraine on the Kiev tramway, 3 foot 5 and $\frac{7}{8}$ inches used in 1911 in Poland on the Częstochowa–Herby line.

Count the Sheep

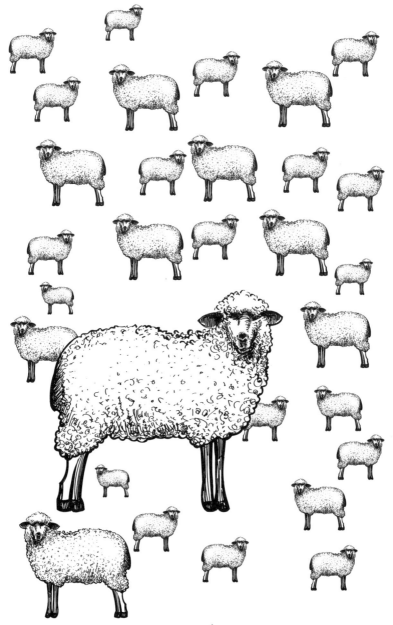

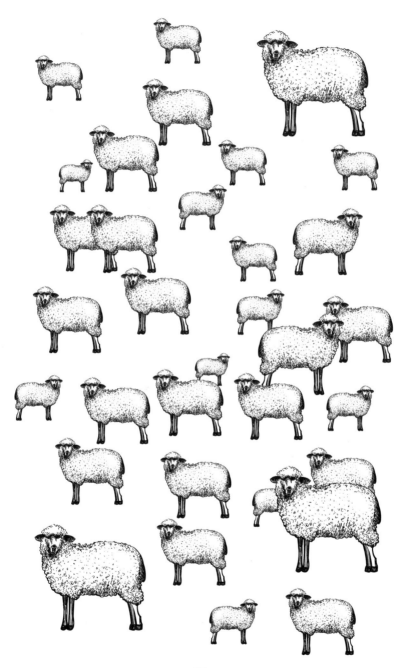

The Dullest Entries in Interesting Diaries

Christopher Columbus
Saturday, Aug. 4th 1492

Steered S.W. by S

President Harry S. Truman
March 3 1947

Spend a pleasant day.
Go to bed and get called at 2:30 A.M. Tuesday.
It is a nice morning. But we run into
clouds over Texas and Oklahoma.

Samuel Pepys
June 17th 1660 (partial transcript)

Lay long abed . . .

Ludwig Wittgenstein
April 10th 1934

Sat watching clouds drift slowly past
the window. Then fell asleep.

George Orwell
September 2nd 1938

Fine & fairly warm.

General Joseph W. Stilwell
Aug 1st 1943

Office in A.M. Usual stuff. P.M. nap.
Read in evening. Good rest.

THE DICTIONARY OF DULLNESS

APATHY, *noun*; inaction due to indifference, lack of enthusiasm, lethargy

DETACHMENT, *noun*; an absence of connection, engagement or interest

DOLDRUMS, *noun*; a place or period of stagnation, ennui or lassitude

DULLNESS, *noun*; the property of being boring, tedious or uninteresting

ENNUI, *noun*; a state of boredom, often induced by tedium and a general sense of pointlessness

FATIGUE, *noun*; tiredness, exhaustion, lethargy, sleepiness

FLATNESS, *noun*; a lack of significant or engaging features, a feeling of pointlessness and boredom

INDIFFERENCE, *noun*; a lack of interest, engagement, connection, concern or enthusiasm

LASSITUDE, *noun*; a condition of weary lethargy

LETHARGY, *noun*; a condition of fatigue, emotional inertia, heaviness or indifference

LISTLESSNESS, *noun*; a lack of energy; weariness and sleepy indolence

MONOTONY, *noun*; an absence of variety, the tedium of endless repetition

POCOCURANTISM, *noun*; indifference, carelessness, lethargic lack of interest

SAMENESS, *noun*; a soporific lack of variety; monotony

TAEDIUM VITAE, *noun*; a state of extreme lethargy, boredom of everything

TEDIOUSNESS, *noun*; see TEDIUM

TEDIUM, *noun*; dullness, monotony, boredom, etc.

Get to Sleep

How the Pyramids Were Built

The Egyptian pyramids are pyramid-shaped structures in Egypt. There are over 100 pyramids, mostly built in sandy areas of the desert. For centuries scientists have speculated as to how the pyramids were built. Now we can reveal the true story of the construction process.

Firstly, detailed plans for the pyramids were drawn up by the architects. Then the plans were given to the builders, whose job it was to follow the instructions. A single block of stone was dragged laboriously across the sandy desert and placed in the correct position. Then another single block of stone was dragged slowly across the sand and placed next to the first block, as instructed in the plans. After that, a third block of stone was dragged gradually across the sand, and manoeuvred inch by inch carefully into place, next to the second block, which was still next to the first block, where it had been positioned. After this a fourth block was dragged slowly across the sand and inched carefully into its correct position. And then a fifth block was dragged carefully across the sand and moved laboriously into the correct position. These blocks were the first five blocks in either the external wall or the internal structure of the pyramids. The eventual aim was to create a pyramid shape within which there were chambers and tunnels as well as internal structures built out of blocks. So the internal structures needed a base block as well as the external walls.

When the first line of blocks of stone was as long as the plans had indicated, the builders carefully dragged another block of stone slowly across the sand under the baking hot sun. This would have been a very slow process, with the block only moving a few inches forwards at a time. This block was placed next to the existing line of blocks of stone, but instead of extending the line in either direction, this block was moved slowly and carefully into position adjacent to the line, creating the first element of a perpendicular wall. Then a second block was carefully dragged across the sand and positioned laboriously next to the block that had previously been carefully positioned according to the plans. After this a third block was dragged ever so slowly across the sand. This third block of the new section of the base of the pyramid was placed precisely in position, adjacent to the previous block which had been placed against the first block of the new section, perpendicular to the previous section of the base. This was all, of course, in accordance with the detailed plans which the builders would have been consulting on a regular basis. One block positioned in an incorrect location could have been disastrous. Indeed, had this third block of the new section been positioned wrongly they might have had to carefully drag every one of the previous blocks back across the sand so that they could start all over again.

Eventually, every block in the base layer of the pyramid was correctly and carefully positioned. Laborious though this stage of the construction had been, the next stage was to be even more complex. Now the first block of the second layer had to be dragged slowly and carefully across the desert floor, in the burning heat of the sun, and then laboriously raised up so that it could be placed in the correct position on top of the existing layer of blocks of stone. After that the second block was dragged slowly and carefully across the sand and raised slowly, inch by inch, up to its correct position next to the first block in the second layer of blocks in the pyramid. This block had to be carefully levered up and then manoeuvred into position. Of course, our explanation of this process may not be entirely accurate. Some of the slow careful dragging of blocks across the sand might have been taking place at the same time as the blocks for the layers were being laboriously dragged and cautiously raised into position before the process continued.

T

HE

EYE CHART

OPTICIANS USE IS

CALLED A SNELLEN CHART

IT IS NAMED AFTER HERMAN

SNELLEN WHO CREATED THE FIRST

SUCH CHART IN 1862 THE CHARTS

ARE GENERALLY PRINTED WITH ELEVEN

LINES OF LETTERS IN THE FIRST LINE

THERE WILL BE ONE VERY LARGE LETTER THE

ROWS HAVE INCREASING NUMBERS OF LETTERS AS YOU

GO DOWN THE PAGE, WITH THE LETTERS AT AN INCREASINGLY

SMALL SIZE WHEN YOU TAKE A TEST YOU SIT 6 METRES FROM

THE CHART AND TRY TO READ THE LETTERS ALOUD SNELLEN REGARDED

'STANDARD VISION' AS BEING ABLE TO RECOGNISE ONE OF HIS OPTOTYPES (THE TECHNICAL

NAME FOR THE LETTERS USED IN THE SNELLEN TEST) WITH 5 MINUTES OF ARC. MEANING

THE PERSON CAN DISCRIMINATE A SPATIAL PATTERN WHICH IS DIVIDED BY A VISUAL ANGLE OF ONE MINUTE

OF ARC IN MANY CASES THE SNELLEN TEST HAS NOW BEEN REPLACED BY THE LOGMAR CHART WHICH ALSO USES ROWS

OF LETTERS AND WAS DEVELOPED AT THE NATIONAL VISION RESEARCH INSTITUTE OF AUSTRALIA IN 1976 THE LOGMAR CHART

ALLOWS OPTICIANS TO ATTAIN A GREATER DEGREE OF ACCURACY THAN THE SNELLEN TEST IN ESTIMATING VISUAL ACUITY . . .

A Few Facts about Roundabouts

- The world's first roundabout (in the modern style) was the Brautwiesenplatz in Görlitz, Germany, opened in 1899.

- Columbus Circle in New York, designed by William Phelps Eno, was another early example of a roundabout, from 1904.

- There was also a gyratory system in use for traffic in the Place de l'Étoile in Paris in 1907.

- The first British roundabout (in the modern style) was built in Letchworth Garden City in 1909.

- Roundabouts were first introduced in Australia during the 1950s.

- A 1998 survey in USA towns in which roundabouts had been proposed found 68 per cent of the public opposed them.

- The Danish word for roundabout is *rundkørsel*. The Hungarian word is *körforgalom*.

- The mini-roundabout was invented by Frank Blackmore, of the UK's Transport and Road Research Laboratory.

- In the Channel Islands there are some roundabouts for which neither the cars on the roundabout nor those approaching it have the right of way.

- In the city of Nelson in New Zealand there is an average of one accident on a roundabout per year.

- To build a three-lane roundabout you need a circular space of approximately 67 metres by 91 metres in diameter.

- A raindrop roundabout is a roundabout that isn't round, but is instead shaped like a raindrop.

- As a general rule, when driving on the left, traffic flows clockwise, but when driving on the right, traffic flows counterclockwise.

- There are more than 20,000 roundabouts in France.

- Roundabouts were not introduced in Japan until 2013.

- In some areas of America roundabouts are known as rotaries.

- In certain countries, including Belgium, Poland and Slovenia, a variation on the traditional two-lane roundabout design is known as the turbo roundabout.

- There are over 40 roundabouts in Redditch (near Birmingham in the United Kingdom).

A History of the Post Office
in Indonesia

The current post office organisation in Indonesia is known as Pos Indonesia. It has a fascinating history. The first postage stamp in what was then known as the Dutch East Indies was issued on 1 April 1864. It had a picture of King Willem III of the Netherlands, and the face value was ten cents. Subsequent stamp designs showed further pictures of the Dutch royal family in either one or two colours. In this period the stamps were mostly printed in the Netherlands by the firm of Joh. Enschedé Haarlem. However, there were also stamps printed locally by Reproductie drijf Topografische dienst. The early postal service was called Post-Telegraaf- en Telefoondienst. This is Dutch for the post, telegraph and telephone service. This version of the Indonesian postal service was initially established in 1906. It remained in operation for 49 years. It was widely referred to as PTT (which is an acronym for Post- Telegraaf- en Telefoondienst).

After the Second World War the central post office in Bandung was taken into state control following the declaration of independence by the newly named Indonesia. Renamed the Indonesia Post Administration, the first stamp was issued in 1946 and showed a cow and the Indonesian flag. It was printed in Yogyakarta in two colours. In 1954 the stamp-printing process was transferred to the new local printer Pertjetakan Kebajoran. The PTT was responsible for distributing the stamps to every post office in the country. Stamps in this period depicted themes including agriculture, industry, social welfare, rural development, politics and transportation. People who featured on subsequent stamps included Sukarno, the first President of Indonesia, as well as Indonesian heroes such as Abdul Muis, Sultan Hasanuddin, Suryopranoto, Teungku Cik di Tiro, Tuanku Imam Bonjol, Teuku Umar, K. H. Samanhudi,

Kapitan Pattimura, K. H. Ahmad Dahlan, Sisingamangaraja XII and Ki Hajar Dewantara.

The PTT was converted into a state-owned company in 1961. In 1965 it was divided into two separate companies. One focused on telecommunication while the other focused on mail. The mail services company was subsequently reorganised in 1978 and renamed as Pos Indonesia in 1995. Pos Indonesia operates in 11 regional divisions across the country. The first number of an area's postal code indicates which region an address is in. The next two digits identify the city or region. The fourth digit identifies the district in more detail, while the fifth digit indicates the specific place.

A postal code starting with 1 is in Jakarta, Banten or West Java. A code starting with 2 is in Aceh, North Sumatra, West Sumatra, Riau or the Riau Islands. A 3 indicates Bengkulu, Jambi, Bangka-Belitung, South Sumatra or Lampung. A 4 indicates Banten or West Java (in different areas to the areas covered by the 1 codes). A 5 indicates Central Java or Yogyakarta, and a 6 indicates East Java. Up to this point the postal codes are more or less identical to the first 6 of the 11 regional divisions of the post office (Pos Indonesia) but, interestingly, the postal codes only go up to the number 9, while there are 11 regions. The reasons for this difference between the postal codes and the regional divisions are complex – in order to explain it we will need to consider the organisation of the post office in more detail.

Each region operates 200 or more sub-regions. These range from inner city and outer city, to towns and villages in the countryside. The country also contains 17,000 islands that can only be reached by sea or by air. There are 3,700 post offices in the country in total. The reason why the numbers of the regions don't match up with the numbers used in the postal codes is partly to do with the size of the regional divisions.

Spot the Difference

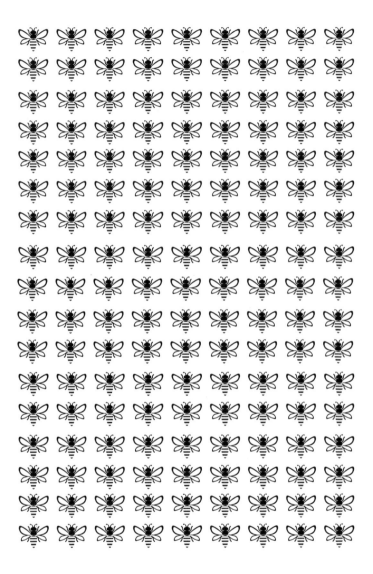

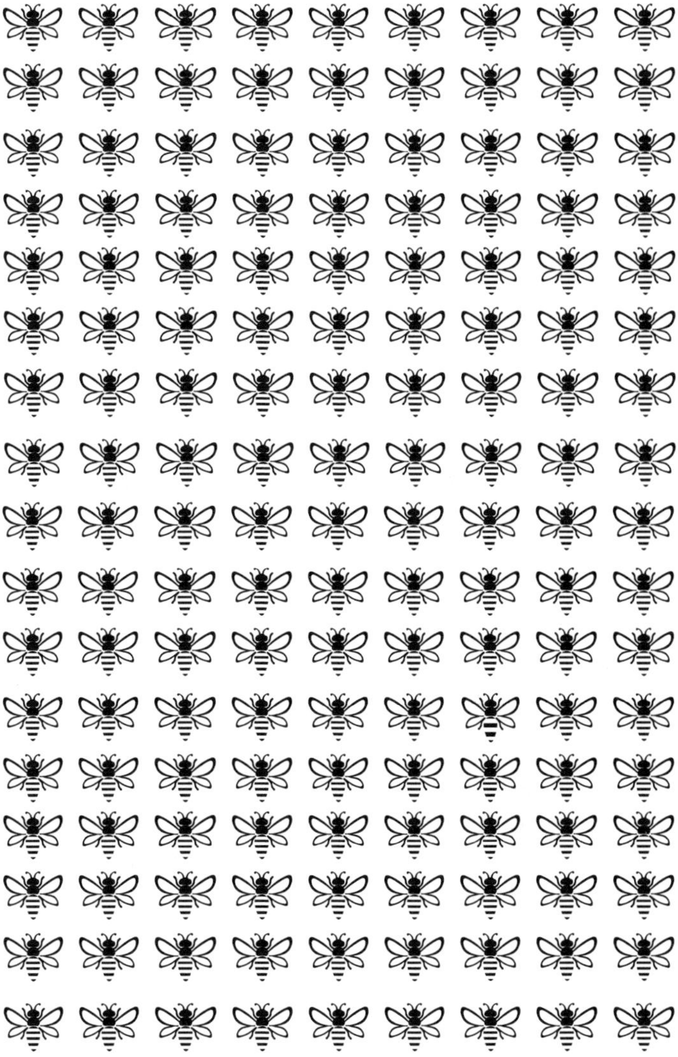

An Interesting Number Theorem Debunked

The Interesting Number Theorem is an interesting theorem from the field of number theory, which is the part of mathematics that deals with the theory of numbers. The Theorem works through a process of *reductio ad absurdum*. This is a Latin term for imagining that something is true in order to prove that it isn't true. Mathematicians are fond of imagining things that are not true. For instance, when they needed to pretend that there is a square root of -1 they imagined the number called i. If you multiply i by itself the product is -1, even though i doesn't actually exist. In order to make this clear, mathematicians refer to multiples of i as imaginary numbers. This is to distinguish them from non-imaginary numbers which also don't exist in the physical world, but which can be represented in the physical world. For this representation, mathematicians often refer to something which is known as Zermelo–Fraenkel Set Theory. This is an interesting theory that uses sets as the basis of all mathematics. A set is a collection of things. What kind of things they are doesn't really matter. They can be imaginary things or real things, but either way we are going to imagine that we have a set of them, and the number of things in the set is equivalent to the number we might use to represent them. So sets are a kind of a representation of numbers, which are a representational construct, used to count things in the real world, but which are also useful for counting imaginary things. If we want to represent zero, for instance, we imagine an empty set, or nothingness. It's hard to imagine a set that contains i things, but that doesn't matter because we can construct a set with one member, then imagine that set being subtracted from nothing, and then imagine finding the square root of something that is less than nothing.

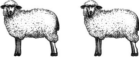

So having established some interesting facts about real and imaginary numbers and ways of representing such numbers using Zermelo–Fraenkel Set Theory, we can move on to the next question: what is the Interesting Number Theorem? Essentially, the question here is whether some numbers are more interesting than other numbers. The answer to this is fairly obvious to a mathematician. It's self-evident that 341 is more interesting than 66, or that 4095 is more interesting than 2491, for instance. And 253 is more interesting than 611. A quirky little number such as 42 might be seen as more interesting than 97, though that is obviously a slightly more controversial suggestion. Also, 1722 is extremely interesting, but there isn't very much that is interesting about 171 at all: that certainly seems like a pretty boring number and many mathematicians would concur.

So the next question that mathematicians like to imagine someone asking is whether there are any numbers that are simply uninteresting. If there are then we could call such numbers boring. There would then be a set of boring numbers and a finite or infinite number that could be associated with that set depending on whether the set of boring numbers was finite or infinite. To a mathematician, it's obvious that the next question has to be, 'What is the smallest boring number?' At this point there is an interesting problem. Zero is a number. As we've seen, in order to represent zero we have to imagine nothingness. Imagine an empty space, in which there are no objects. Is that interesting? Imagine a snowy day but with no snowflakes. Imagine a desert without any sand. Imagine no raindrops, no sky, no sounds, nothing whatsoever. Imagine a long motorway stretching out into the distance, with no cars, no verge, no bridges, no horizon. Imagine a beach with no pebbles. Imagine the infinite vastness of space, with no stars, no planets, no comets, no particles of any sort. This is the empty set, the null set, the void, an imaginary representation of nothingness without end.

Some Facts about Canals

- In 1816 there were only 100 miles of canals in the United States of America.

- The Dessel–Turnhout–Schoten Canal across the province of Antwerp in Belgium is 63 kilometres long.

- In the French canal system the canal that has the least overhead clearance at bridges is the Canal du Nivernais, for which vessels must have less than 2.9 metres clearance above the water.

- When President James Madison vetoed the federal works bill in March 1817 there was a temporary slowdown in the building of the Erie Canal until more funds were secured.

- In 1798 Napoleon intended to build a canal across the Suez Isthmus. But then he changed his mind.

- Ireland's Royal Canal was once mentioned in a poem by Brendan Behan.

- Water in the Vlakfontein Canal in South Africa flows at approximately 5.7 cubic metres per second.

- The Havel Canal in Germany is one of three separate canals that have both their starting point and finishing point on the River Havel.

- Qibao is one of several well-known 'water towns' in close proximity to Shanghai. However, it doesn't have any canals.

- The Schulz Canal in Nundah is the only canal in Queensland, Australia.

- The shortest canal in England is the Wardle Lock Branch of the Trent and Mersey Canal. It consists a few yards of canal on either side of a 72-foot-long lock.

- In 1841 there were 19 steamboats operating on the Rideau Canal in Canada.

- There are no canals on the island of Guadalcanal.

- The Ohau A power station in New Zealand is supplied with water by two canals: one from Lake Pukaki and one from Lake Ohau.

The History of Gravel

To a geologist, gravel is any loose rock that is larger than 2 millimetres in its longest dimension but no more than about 60 millimetres. Gravel is simply rock that is within this specific particle size range. Larger rocks are gradually eroded into smaller rocks and this leads to the formation of natural gravel deposits. However, gravel can also be made by mechanically crushing rocks. Many roads and paths have a gravel surface, especially in low-traffic rural areas. It may also be used as an aggregate in concrete. There are more roads in the world that have a gravel surface than a concrete or tarmac one. There are more than 400,000 kilometres of gravel-surfaced roads in Russia. Rock particles smaller than gravel are geologically classified as sand. Rock particles larger than gravel and pebble are geologically classified as cobble. The erosion caused by rivers and waves tends to pile up gravel in large quantities. This can lead to the gravel becoming compacted into sedimentary rock, which geologists call conglomerate. Quarries where gravel is extracted are called gravel pits. There are many types of gravel. They include: bank gravel, which is naturally deposited gravel adjacent to rivers and streams and which is also known as bank run or river run; bench gravel, which is a layer of gravel on the side of a valley left over from when the stream lower down the valley was at a higher level; crushed stone, which refers to gravel that has been crushed and mixed with a blend of stones which, when used on roads and driveways, sometimes has tar imposed on it; fine gravel, which is gravel that is only 2 millimetres to 4 millimetres in its longest dimension; lag gravel, which is a surface accumulation of coarse gravel left behind after the removal of fine gravel; and pea gravel, which is a type of gravel consisting of small rounded stones used in concrete surfaces.

White Noise: a Technical Explanation

White noise is created by generating a random signal made up of serially uncorrelated random variables that has the same intensity at many different frequencies. To be precise, the variable is not entirely random as the bandwidth is bounded by the actual physical mechanism that is used to generate the noise. The range of audible sound frequencies stretches from 20 to 20,000 hertz. A randomly generated sample of white noise in this bounded area sounds like a hissing noise.

We tend to hear white noise as having more high-frequency content than low, even though the actual generation process involves randomly generating noise at all frequencies. This is because each octave has twice as many frequencies as the one below it. From 100 hertz to 200 hertz there are 100 discrete frequencies. The next octave, from 200 hertz to 400 hertz, contains twice as many frequencies as that. The octave after that contains 400 discrete frequencies. The octave after that contains 800 frequencies and so on. In order to combat this issue, you can instead generate 'pink noise', in which some of the higher frequencies are damped down in order to generate a noise that seems more consistent across the full range of frequencies.

It is important to understand how the random variables that define the frequencies on which noise is generated are derived. It is sometimes incorrectly stated that white noise is the same thing as Gaussian noise. Gaussian noise is made up of a random signal, in much the same way as white noise is. However, Gaussian noise follows the normal statistical distribution (also known as Gaussian distribution or the bell curve), as suggested by the name. Gaussian noise sounds similar to white noise but the two are not necessarily identical. The random generation of the frequencies in standard white noise need not follow the normal distribution.

Any given random vector, meaning a process that produces vectors of real numbers following a process that is not fully determinate, can be described as white noise if it has a probability distribution with no mean, a finite variance and statistically uncorrelated components. For the components to be statistically uncorrelated it is necessary that they have a covariance of zero. (Covariance is a statistical measure of how correlated the variance of two variables are, in other words how the variance of the variables varies. The more correlated the variance of the variables, the more positive the covariance value will be. Two variables with negative covariance are variables that tend to vary in opposite directions.) Neither a positive nor negative covariance should be shown by the variables that make up true white noise. The variance of the variables should not vary, and they should have a covariance of zero.

If you want Gaussian white noise, rather than other types of white noise, you would also need each of the variables to have a normal distribution, as well as a zero mean. You would also need each of the variables to have the exact same variance. Note that it is also possible to generate white noise with different types of statistical distribution. For instance, you can use a Poisson distribution or a Cauchy distribution.

Some people use white noise in order to help them sleep. Science suggests that it is not actual noises in the night that wake you up, but changes in frequency. Since white noise consists of continuous noise at every frequency, an additional noise on top of white noise will not consist of a particular change in frequency. So a consistent background of white noise will damp down any extraneous noises and allow for more consistent levels of sleep, with less variance and variability in the consistency.

A World Almanac of Pine Cones

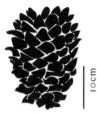

COULTER PINE

VERY HEAVY

KNOB CONE PINE

VERY HARD

JEFFREY PINE

NOT VERY SPIKY

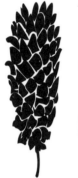

SUGAR PINE

VERY LONG

PONDEROSA PINE

VERY PRICKLY

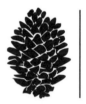

LODGEPOLE PINE

VERY TINY

PINYON PINE

VERY EDIBLE

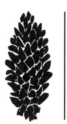

LIMBER PINE

VERY THICK

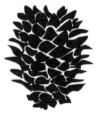

HICKORY PINE

VERY HARDY

Some Minor European Politicians

- In the Belgian government of 2014, the Secretary of State for Administrative Simplification was Theo Francken.

- In the seventh government of the Republic of Croatia, elected in 2000, the Minister for Crafts, Small and Mid-sized Entrepreneurship was Željko Pecek.

- In the 1993–4 government of Ireland, the Minister for Education was Niamh Bhreathnach.

- In the Belarus government of 2016, the head of the subordinate agency called the Republican Centre for Sanatorium-and-Spa Treatment was Gennady Bolbatovsky.

- In the 1867–8 Romanian cabinet, there were two Ministers of the Interior: Ştefan Golescu and Ion C. Brătianu.

- In the German cabinet from 1991 to 1994, the Minister for Post and Communications was Christian Schwarz-Schilling.

- In the government of the Republic of Abkhazia, Nerses Nersesyan was appointed in 2005 as Minister of Standards, Metrology and Certification.

- In the Czech Republic, in the government formed in 2007, there were two ministers without portfolio who had the same surname: Cyril Svoboda and Pavel Svoboda.

- In the 2016 cabinet of Montenegro, Suzana Pribilović had the role of Minister of Public Administration.

- Andrus Ansip's third cabinet in Estonia (formed in 2005) was a coalition between the Estonian Reform Party and the Pro Patria and Res Publica Union. The Minister of Regional Affairs was Siim Valmar Kiisler.

- In the 2015 Finnish government, the appointee for the Minister of Transport and Communications was Anne Berner.

- In the Swedish government of 1996, Leif Pagrotsky had two portfolios, serving both as the Minister for Nordic Cooperation and also as the Minister for Foreign Trade.

- In France, the Ministry of Budget, Public Accounts and Civil Administration of France was created in 2007. The first minister was Éric Woerth.

Fog and Mist:
a Scientific Exposition

If you've ever wondered what it is like to be inside a cloud, the closest direct experience you are likely to have comes in the form of fog and mist. Fog is formed in exactly the same way as clouds – as a mass of cloud-water droplets or ice crystals suspended in the air. The main differences between fog and cloud are that fog is found close to ground level and is generally formed through ground and wind conditions in the immediate area, from surrounding areas of water or moist ground. (Fog and mist are only distinguished by how dense the water droplets are in the air – most attempts to differentiate them are based on visibility.)

In the same way as for clouds, fog develops when water droplets condense onto tiny particles in the air. This is why fog tends to be thicker in industrial areas with high pollution levels – because there are more particulates in the air which can act as condensation nuclei. Once the water droplets condense, they remain dispersed in the air. Fog is a colloid, which is the scientific name for a mixture, of gas and liquid in this case, in which the dispersed substance is denser than a solution, but not as dense as a suspension.

Different types of fog are named after the particular ways in which the air can become sufficiently saturated with water vapour and cool enough for condensation to occur. Radiation fog is most common in autumn and winter, and occurs when the ground cools during the night because of thermal radiation (especially when the sky is relatively cloud-free). This leads to condensation in the air immediately above the ground and, in calm conditions, to a thin layer of fog, which will disperse soon after sunrise. (In this form it can also be referred to as ground fog.) However, wind turbulence can churn this up into a thicker layer, which may persist for much longer at altitude or in areas bounded by high ground. Advection fog is caused by moist air being blown by winds over cool surfaces, leading to condensation and thus to cloud droplets. It is most common over snowy or icy land or cool areas of the sea. Upslope fog occurs when a body of air flows across an upward slope and will tend to form further up the slope rather than at the bottom of the slope. However, the fog formed upslope can gradually seep back down the slope into the lower areas. It can look like a cloud or fog depending on whether you are standing in it or below it. That which flows from an upslope down into a valley can be called valley fog. Steam fog forms when water vapour mixes with cold air and the vapour condenses into fog. You can spot this when wisps of fog resembling steam rise up from the surface of a lake or an ocean. It is most likely to happen in situations where the water is warm and the air is cold. The fog rises upwards and becomes more and more dense, leading to reduced visibility and dampness. Frontal fog is a type of fog found in frontal zones and frontal passages. There are three types of frontal fog: warm-front pre-frontal fog; cold-front post-frontal fog; and frontal-passage fog. The first two types, pre-frontal and post-frontal fog, are caused by rain falling into cold air with the result that the dew point is raised. Frontal-passage fog happens in a variety of other situations in which damp cold air masses mix with air at a variety of different temperatures. Look out of the window. Imagine that mist is gradually forming in the area, rising up from the ground, obscuring first the ground and then more and more of the landscape around you. The mist is gradually getting thicker, turning into a dense fog. Everything you can see is gradually disappearing, fading into nothingness. There is nothing to see here.

The Taxonomy of Micromoths

The microlepidoptera (micromoths) are a non-monophyletic grouping of families of moth. As it is a non-monophyletic grouping, micromoth enthusiasts generally use the property of smallness as a way of identifying micromoths. Moths with a wingspan of less than 20mm qualify as micromoths. Because they are very small they can be quite hard to identify using external phenotypic markings. (Some are so small that they are quite hard to see in the first place.)

Efforts to more clearly define the term *micromoth* have proven inadequate, so the controversy will continue over which categories of moth should be included in the microlepidoptera and which should be included in the macrolepidoptera. There are 30 main groups that are generally acknowledged to be microlepidoptera. These include the Gelechioidea (which include Gelechiidae, Oecophoridae, Lecithoceridae, Cosmopterigidae, Coleophoridae, Elachistidae, Momphidae, Ethmiidae, Blastobasidae and a few other subfamilies), Pyraloidea (including Pyralidae and Crambidae), Tortricidae, Tineoidea (which covers the Tineidae, Eriocottidae, Acrolophidae, Arrhenophanidae, Psychidae and Lypusidae), Gracillarioidea, Nepticuloidea, Yponomeutoidea (which includes Yponomeutidae, Acrolepiidae, Ypsolophidae and Plutellidae) and numerous other groupings.

Some of the groupings that we haven't mentioned yet are distinguished by particular features. The types of moth that fall into the microlepidoptera include sedge moths, sun moths, lyonet moths, plume moths, many-plumed moths, tropical leaf moths, day-flying moths, fairy moths, metalmark moths, mandibulate archaic moths, sparkling archaic sun moths and spring jewel moths.

Economic Statistics from the First Two Five-Year Plans in the Soviet Union

- As a proportion of the land under cultivation, from 1929 to 1933 the area under cultivation for grain grew by less than 6 per cent, while the area under cultivation for the production of vegetables and melons grew by about 13 per cent.

- In 1932 there were 78.4 million hectares in state and collectivised farms, and 21.3 million hectares in individual peasant farms. The following year that had changed to 85.8 million hectares in state and collectivised farms, and 15.7 million hectares in individual peasant farms.

- During the second five-year plan in 1933 there were 50.2 million sheep and goats while in 1934 there were 51.9 million. Over the same two years the number of horses fell from 16.6 million to 15.7 million.

- The total number of tractors in the Soviet Union grew from 148,500 in 1932 to 204,100 in 1933.

- The total volume of industrial output expressed as a percentage of the pre-war level in 1913 was 194.3 per cent in 1929.

- The total output of private industry in 1933 expressed in roubles at the price level of 1926–7 was 28 million in 1933. It was also 28 million in 1937.

- The gross output of consumer goods in 1931 was 15,100 million roubles.

- Oil extraction as a percentage of the total gross output of the economy was 1.8 per cent in 1929, but just 1.4 per cent in 1933.

- The number of state and cooperative retail stores and booths at the end of the year was 286,236 in 1934. This had risen to 289,473 in 1936.

- Between 1936 and 1937 the amount of freight transport measured in millions of tons rose by 31,400 from 323,400 to 354,800. However, in the same time period the amount transported by river fell by 2,200 from 72,300 to 70,100.

- The number of books held in public libraries rose by 47.2 per cent between 1933–4 and 1938–9.

Brownian Motion in Dust Particles

Think about dust particles dancing in the light of a sunbeam. The Roman thinker Lucretius observed this phenomenon and suggested that they were moving that way because of the collisions of millions of tiny atoms. But no one knew what atoms were, only that everything could be broken down into smaller and smaller parts and that the very smallest part that something could be broken down into might be called an atom. This view went back to earlier Greek and Indian philosophers. For instance, Leucippus and Democritus claimed that all existence was made of either atoms or the void. Against this Heraclitus argued that all existence is change. Opposed to this was Parmenides who argued that all change is illusion. He denied the existence of motion, change or anything of interest in existence. Parmenides also claimed there was no such thing as a void because if the void is, then it is not nothing, in which case it isn't the void. Other contemporaries argued that all illusion is a void, or that all emptiness is something, or that something is either always present or never absent and thus never nothing, but their names have mostly been lost to posterity.

The motion of dust particles in the air has many parallels in other observable phenomena. In 1785 Jan Ingenhousz described the irregular motion of coal dust particles on the surface of alcohol. In 1827 Robert Brown described this kind of motion in particles of pollen in the water. His observation led to the description of such activity as Brownian motion. Brownian motion can also be observed in the diffusion of coloured dye in a liquid or in colloidal particles in a variety of experimental settings. The best way to describe Brownian motion is to imagine a tiny particle of something in a liquid or gas. As you try to focus on this tiny particle, it keeps darting around in random different directions. No matter how hard you stare at this tiny, tiny particle, you can't predict which way it will dart next.

Brownian motion is best understood as a stochastic process. This essentially means it is an accumulation of tiny random events. Each event can be predicted using a probabilistic model. So the tiny particle that we are straining our eyes to watch is behaving in a probabilistic manner. One way to model such motion is using a Wiener process, which is a continuous-time stochastic process. This in turn is a type of Lévy process (a stochastic process with stationary, independent increments). When we model a stochastic process in this way, we are creating a representation of the motion of a tiny particle whose repetitive, random movements are unpredictable. Of course, unpredictability does not prevent us from creating a probabilistic model, so long as we understand that the modelling remains purely stochastic.

When we are mathematically modelling the Brownian motion of tiny particles in sunlight (or in a liquid or any other gaseous substance) it can be useful to use the concept of a Brownian bridge (which is a continuous-time stochastic with a probability distribution that can be derived from a Wiener process). We can also supplement this method of modelling with tests such as the Kolmogorov–Smirnov test, which is a non-parametric test of the relative values of one-dimensional probability distributions that are continuous rather than non-continuous, and the Glivenko–Cantelli theorem, which determines the asymptotic behaviour of the empirical distribution function. However, before we return to the problem of trying to guess which way a tiny particle will move next, we need further to consider the issue of how Brownian motion relates to Gaussian distribution and to a further digression on the subject of the Pre-Socratic atomists and their opponents regarding issues of change, motion, something, nothingness and the void.

The Drying of Paint: a Technical Explanation

When describing the drying process of paint, we need to start with a detailed understanding of the chemical composition of the average paint. This is firstly made up of pigments, which give the paint its colour and opacity, and some kind of binder or resin, by which we mean a polymer, which creates the chemical structure that contains the pigment. In addition the paint will need an extender, which introduces some larger pigment particles that strengthen the mixture and reduce the need for binder, as well as an organic solvent or water which will reduce the viscosity of the paint and a variety of other additives. The additives might include dispersants, which give an orderly structure to the particles of pigment, silicones to make the chemical composition more robust, thixotropic agents, which modify the texture of the paint when the brush is applied to it, anti-settling agents and such things as bactericides, fungicides or algaecides. Crucially, the additives may also include driers, which are drying agents that can affect how long the paint takes to dry.

There are different factors that affect different types of paint. Firstly, let's take a look at the drying of water-based paint. This happens in two main phases: evaporation and coalescence. Evaporation happens when water molecules from the mixture gradually evaporate along with other volatile liquids that are contained within the chemical composition of the paint. Some of these liquids will evaporate faster than others so, as long as it is wet, the remaining mixture of the paint will be in a process of flux in which the proportion of first water and then other volatile liquids is falling at a constant or non-constant rate. Following the evaporation phase of the drying process we enter into the coalescence phase, in which the separate particles of the polymer binder, which we have already noted as being part of the chemical composition of the paint, start to coalesce with each other into a solid film or shield.

How Many Peas in a Pod?

- How many peas you should expect to find in a pea pod depends on the variety of pea, but, on average, green peas have six to seven peas in the pod.

- Unusual pea pods can contain anything from two to twenty peas.

- Three metres of green peas should usually yield more than 90 kilograms of shelled peas, depending on the weather, soil, variety selected and frequency of harvest.

- To maximise yield, peas should be picked every three to four days.

- If a pod matures to the point where the peas are viable as seed, the plant will die, so the peas must be picked before they mature.

- Planting can take place when the soil temperature reaches 10 degrees centigrade, but plants grow best at temperatures of 14 to 18 degrees centigrade so this is the best temperature for maximising the number of peas in a pod.

- The green pea that we most often eat is the seed of the pod fruit *Pisum sativum*.

- Pea pods are technically fruit because they are containers for seeds and grow from the ovary of a pea flower.

- The average pea weighs between a tenth and a third of a gram.

- Peas have both low-growing and vining cultivars, but the tip of a climber does not affect the number of peas in the pod.

- Pea plants are self-pollinators, which means they pollinate themselves.

- The earliest archaeological finds that show evidence of the consumption of peas date from the late Neolithic era in areas that are now part of Greece, Syria and Egypt. The varieties of pea consumed were similar to the peas consumed today, with a similar number of peas in each pod.

- Peas were also being grown in Georgia in the fifth millennium BC.

- There is evidence of pea growing in Afghanistan (2000 BC), and in Pakistan and India (2250–1750 BC).

A History of Pottery-Making

Pottery is one of the oldest human inventions. It was already being manufactured by the Neolithic period. Gravettian figurines such as those excavated at Dolní Věstonice in the Czech Republic, including the famous Venus of Dolní Věstonice, a statuette of a female nude, may date back to as long ago as 29,300 BC.

The earliest vessels made out of pottery have been dated at approximately 18,000 BC or possibly 18,100 BC. They were found in a cave in China. They were most likely used for the purpose of cookery. Early pottery vessels dating from approximately 16,000 BC have also been excavated from another cave in China. Vessels found in the Amur River basin in Russia are from about 2,000 years later. Excavations at a site in Japan in 1998 have uncovered earthenware fragments which have been dated as early as 14,500 or 14,750 BC, which places them in the Jōmon period. Jōmon means 'marked with cord' in Japanese. This is due to the fact that there are markings made on the vessels using sticks and cords in the process of manufacture. In Africa pottery manufacturing was in existence by the 10th millennium BC, as pottery found there has been dated back to at least 9400 BC. In South America pottery has been found from the same approximate period. Pottery from the same period has also been found in East Asia.

Early forms of pottery were made in open fires in which the clay could be baked at relatively low temperatures. The items made out of pottery would be formed by hand and wouldn't at this time be glazed or decorated. A relatively short baking time was used, in which the temperatures in the fire could be relatively high, up to 800 or 900 degrees centigrade. Early potters used clay that could be easily found in their region. Common red clay was a common source for pottery in the early period. However, the drawback of red clay was that when it was baked it tended to be permeable to liquids.

As a general rule, early pieces of pottery were made with rounded bottoms because the pottery was more breakable and fragile than modern pottery, and it was important to avoid sharp edges. Pots would be made through some combination of pinching and coiling. The first actual kilns were trench kilns, which can also be called pit kilns, which were holes dug in the ground in which a fire could be made.

Pit kilns and trench kilns were better insulated from wind and thus easier to control and to achieve consistently high temperatures in. The next innovation was the potter's wheel which was probably invented in Mesopotamia between 6500 and 4100 BC. By this stage of history, pottery was becoming a cottage industry in which a potter or group of potters would work to create pottery for sale or barter. More and more different types of pottery started to become available as the potters became more skilled at their craft. Vessels were made to store, carry, stand, support, decorate and contain things.

The process of glazing was probably first employed in China sometime between the thirteenth and fifteenth centuries BC. It was only possible to glaze pots once potters used kilns that could achieve higher temperatures. The art of decorating pottery has gradually evolved since then with a wider variety of glazes and other forms of decoration coming into wider use. Minoan pottery of the early period, for instance, used complex painted forms of decoration that featured a variety of themes from nature and elsewhere. Porcelain was first manufactured during the Tang Dynasty in China (AD 618–906). Porcelain was subsequently made in Korea and there are examples of porcelain from Japan in the late sixteenth century. Those countries had supplies of kaolin on which the process of making porcelain depended heavily. Porcelain was not made outside East Asia until the eighteenth century.

47

Comparative Lengths of
Airport Runways

A number of factors affect the length of airport runways. Larger aircraft require longer runways, since it takes them longer to reach the speed of 150 to 180 mph that is required for take-off. The take-off weight and the power of the aircraft's engines are also significant. At high elevations and high temperatures the low air pressure makes it harder to achieve take-off, so longer runways are required. Low air pressure also affects the power that the aircraft's engines can achieve.

Some of the longest airport runways in the world are in China and Russia. Qamdo Bamda Airport and Shigatse Peace Airport in China, as well as Ramenskoye Airport and Ulyanovsk Vostochny Airport in Russia all have runways of 5,000 metres or longer.

Runways with lengths of between 4,500 metres and 5,000 metres include Embraer Unidade Gavião Peixoto Airport in Brazil, Upington Airport in South Africa, Hamad International Airport in Qatar, Madrid–Torrejón Airport in Spain, Erbil International Airport in Iraq, Bole International Airport in Egypt, N'djili Airport in the Democratic Republic of the Congo and Windhoek Hosea Kutako International Airport in Namibia.

Iran alone has ten airports that have runways between the length of 4,000 metres and 4,500 metres. These are Bushehr Airport, Isfahan International Airport, Shiraz International Airport, Hamadan Air Base, Zahedan Airport, Dayrestan Airport, Tehran Imam Khomeini International Airport, Omidiyeh Air Base, Shahid Sadooghi Airport and Mehrabad Airport. In the same range of runway length of 4,000 to 4,500 metres there is one airport in Burma, one in Canada, two in China, one in Ecuador, one in France, four in India, one in each of Indonesia, Israel, Kenya, Kyrgyzstan, Libya, Malaysia, Mexico, Morocco, Peru and Somalia, two in Saudi Arabia, one in South Africa, three in the United Arab Emirates and more than twenty in the United States of America.

At the opposite extreme, there are some runways as short as 400 metres. Matekane Air Strip in Lesotho, for instance, is 400 metres. At Out Skerries in Shetland there is a runway that is just 364 metres. There are numerous other short runways in the Scottish islands. Papa Westray, Fair Isle and Stronsay all have runways of less than 550 metres. Juancho E. Yrausquin Airport on the island of Saba also has a short runway that is just 400 metres.

Some of the airports that have a runway length between 500 metres and 1,000 metres are Miquelon Airport in France, Cameta Airport in Brazil, Nuuk Airport in Greenland, Kerema Airport in Papua New Guinea, Kilkenny Airport in Ireland, Roseau Airport in Dominica, Portimão Airport in Portugal, Land's End Airport in England, Castlebar Airport in Ireland, New Nickerie Airport in Surinam, Wexford Airport in Ireland, Baillif Airport in Basse Terre (Guadeloupe), Anatom Airport in Vanuatu, Isles of Scilly Airport in the United Kingdom, Yasawa Airport in Fiji and Courchevel Airport in France.

As well as knowing the length of an airport runway, it is important to know its orientation. For this purpose, runways are given by a number between 01 and 36, to indicate the magnetic azimuth of the runway. A runway numbered 09 points east (90°), runway 18 is south (180°), runway 27 points west (270°) and runway 36 points to the north (360°). If it is landing on or taking off from runway 09, a plane is heading 90° (east). If it is landing on or taking off from runway 18, a plane is heading south (180°). If it is landing on or taking off from runway 27, a plane is heading west (270°). And, of course, when landing on or taking off from runway 36 a plane is heading north (360°).

Portfolio Theory:
an Introduction

Portfolio theory is that body of mathematical and business theory that allows us to calculate such things as the expected return of an investment, and the expected return of a portfolio of investments. It is useful to investors who want to perform such calculations. To calculate the expected return for an individual investment in portfolio theory, we first assess the probability of a range of possible outcomes and assign certain expected values to each of the outcomes by considering a range of variables and the varying results they might influence with respect to the asset.

For each possible outcome we multiply the assessed return by its probability and then find the sum of the results. To calculate the expected return on a portfolio, take the weighted average expected return of the individual assets, as previously calculated through an assessment of the various variables and the sum of the probability of the possible outcomes. Then take the sum of the weighted average expected return of the individual assets. To calculate variance for an individual investment, we return to the assessment of the variables that influence particular possible outcomes and then simply calculate the sum of the squares of the difference between the expected return in a particular possible outcome and the mean expected return, not forgetting of course to weight this calculation by the specific probabilities of the particular possible outcomes, given the probability of the variables that feed into the calculation.

As ever, standard deviation is the square root of the variance.

At this stage we might want to calculate the covariance between two assets over a given period. For this you need to calculate the actual return from each given particular period in the overall period that is under consideration. Then we need to establish the difference between the average return and the actual return by subtracting the former from the latter for each of the particular assets we are attempting to assess. In order to assess the covariance of the assets, we now find the sum of these differences and divide by the number of periods we are assessing for the particular assets. Covariance, of course, is a way of measuring the variation between the variance of the variables we are assessing.

At this point, if we want to assess these assets more assiduously the obvious next step is to find the standard deviation for the entire portfolio. If, for instance, the portfolio we are assessing is made up of only two assets, we need to find the proportion of the portfolio that is invested in the first asset and multiply it by the variance of the first asset (as calculated earlier by assessing the various variables that might affect the variance of the second asset). Then we need to find the proportion of the portfolio that is invested in the second asset and multiply it by the variance of the second asset (as calculated earlier by considering the various variables that might affect the variance of the first asset). We add these together then add a third term which is the product of the weighting of the two assets, the standard deviation of the two assets and the correlation coefficient of the two assets (which we should previously have calculated by dividing the covariance of the two assets by the product of the standard deviation of each asset). The standard deviation of the portfolio is the square root of this particular product.

However, this method of calculation is only useful for a portfolio with two assets. For a portfolio with three or more assets, we start by finding the proportion of the portfolio that is invested in the first asset and multiply it by the variance of the first asset (as calculated earlier by assessing the various variables that might affect the variance of the first asset). Then we need to find the proportion of the portfolio that is invested in the second asset and multiply it by the variance of the various variables.

Why Raindrops Are Different Sizes

On average, a raindrop has a diameter of approximately 0.1 to 4.9 millimetres. There are some exceptions: raindrops of 8 millimetres have been known to occur. Larger sizes of raindrop are rare because at a larger size the particles break up into smaller pieces. There are many factors that contribute to the determination of the diameter or size of a raindrop. The speed at which a raindrop particle falls downwards is proportional to its diameter. Larger particles thus fall faster than smaller ones. (If you drop a cannonball and a smaller ball they will accelerate at the same rate, but with raindrops you have to take into account wind resistance.) The maximum distance a raindrop falls before it evaporates is dependent on the process by which a liquid turns into a gas, which is also proportionate to the size of the drop. As a raindrop falls downwards it meets air resistance. Frictional drag caused by the air molecules increases proportionately to the acceleration of the raindrop. Eventually the forces of friction and gravitation balance out and the raindrop reaches its terminal velocity, which is the velocity with which its fall terminates. Smaller drops don't reach as high a terminal velocity as larger drops. Large raindrops tend to signify a higher level of turbulence in the air and stronger upward draughts or air meeting resistance in the clouds above. Raindrops aren't usually shaped like tears, which is often how people depict them in drawings and other images. Instead, they are oblate spheroids, which look like spheres with a dent, or saucers. A hundred years ago scientists thought the size of a raindrop was determined by forces at work within the cloud before the raindrop falls. More recently it has been shown that raindrops can form or disintegrate many times as they fall. A raindrop occurs when water vapour within a cloud coalesces around tiny particles within the same cloud. The tiny drops remain closely packed together and this means that they tend to coalesce into larger drops.

A Catalogue of Adverse Weather Conditions Encountered in *Wuthering Heights* by Emily Brontë

- Chapter 1: The 'pure bracing ventilation' and 'power of the north wind' (in an explanation of the 'Wuthering' in Wuthering Heights).

- Chapter 2: Misty and cold with a black frost on the bleak hilltop and the 'first feathery flakes of a snow-shower', turning to thick snow later: 'I approached a window to examine the weather. A sorrowful sight I saw: dark night coming down prematurely, and sky and hills mingled in one bitter whirl of wind and suffocating snow.'

- Chapter 3: Gusty wind and thick driving snow: 'the whole hill-back was one billowy, white ocean'.

- Chapter 4: Chilly, housebound.

- Chapter 5: A high wind, wild and stormy.

- Chapter 6: Sufficiently damp for Catherine to lose her shoe in a bog on the windy moor.

- Chapter 7: A shower of rain.

- Chapter 8: Summer rain.

- Chapter 9: 'It was a very dark evening for summer: the clouds appeared inclined to thunder.'

Approaching rain, which arrives in huge drops, followed by violent winds and thunder, of sufficient force to knock a tree down, which falls into the house, causing significant damage.

- Chapter 10: 'Bleak winds and bitter northern skies.'

- Chapter 11: A frosty afternoon, 'the ground bare, and the road hard and dry'.

- Chapter 12: Misty darkness. Windy, with swaying trees.

- Chapter 13: Mild winds followed by chilly, inhospitable darkness.

- Chapter 14: Dreary.

- Chapter 15: A scarcely perceptible wind.

- Chapter 16: Bright and cheerful out of doors (as a counterpoint to the frenzied mourning and exhausted anguish indoors, following the death of Catherine in childbirth).

The Vienna Convention on
Road Signs and Signals

The standardisation of road signs, signals and markings is a matter that has received a great deal of attention over the years. For instance, in the 2005–6 session of the United Nations, Resolution A/RES/60/5 implored nations to adhere to the UN Convention on Road Signs and Signals. The most significicant progress towards this end has come in the shape of the Vienna Convention on Road Signs and Signals. The convention was signed in over 70 countries, mostly in Europe but also in Asia and Africa, and ratified in over 65 countries, including Albania, Bahrain, Belarus, Belgium, Bosnia and Herzegovina, the Central African Republic, Chile, Côte d'Ivoire, Cuba, Cyprus, Czech Republic, the Democratic Republic of the Congo, Estonia, Finland, Georgia, Greece, Guyana, Hungary, India, Iran, Iraq, Italy, Kazakhstan, Kuwait, Kyrgyzstan, Latvia, Liberia, Lithuania, Macedonia, Moldova, Mongolia, Montenegro, Morocco, Netherlands, Nigeria, Norway, Pakistan, Paraguay, Philippines, Poland, Romania, Russia, San Marino, Senegal, Serbia, Seychelles, Sierra Leone, Slovakia, Slovenia, Sri Lanka, Tajikistan, Tunisia, Turkey, Turkmenistan, Ukraine, the United Arab Emirates, Uzbekistan and Vietnam.

The story of the Vienna Convention can be traced back to the 1909 International Convention on Motor Traffic in Paris. This dealt with all aspects of roads and traffic, but gave significant attention to the problem of the international standardisation of road signage and signals. Among the documents presented at the International Convention on Motor Traffic was the League of Nations Special Committee of Enquiry on Road Traffic. Another International Convention on Motor Traffic was held in 1926, but the problem of road signs and signals was not fully addressed on that occasion, so another special convention on the Unification of

Road Signs was held in Geneva in 1931. One reason why America is not currently part of the Vienna Convention lies in the response to the 1926 and 1931 conventions. Rather than accept these, the Pan American Union in Washington instead issued their own Convention on the Regulation of Inter-American Automotive Traffic. In 1948 resolution 147 B (VII) of the United Nations Economic and Social Council was passed in response to the latter convention. It called for a new United Nations Conference on Road and Motor Transport to be convened. This in turn led to the 1949 Convention on Road Traffic and a Protocol on Road Signs and Signals.

In 1966 the United Nations Economic and Social Council issued resolution 1129 (XLI). Certain important points of detail in this document were, however, supplemented and replaced in resolution 1203 (XLII). Also two draft conventions were prepared as a basis for a new conference (E/CONF.56/1 and Addendum.1 and Correction.1 and E/CONF.56/3 and Addendum.1 and Correction.1). This very important convention was scheduled by the Economic and Social Council for the months of October and November in 1968. It was held in Vienna, which is why the resulting convention is called the Vienna Convention on Road Signs and Signals.

The Convention categorises road signs and signals into specific categories. These are: danger warning signs, priority signs, prohibitory or restrictive signs, mandatory signs, information, facilities or service signs, direction, position or indication signs and, finally, any additional panels that might be required in order to communicate information to drivers and other users of vehicles. Examples of danger warning signs include yield signs, stop signs, specific types of priority signs, end priority signs, priority for oncoming traffic signs and priority over oncoming traffic signs. Examples of prohibitory signs include standard prohibitory signs, parking prohibitory signs and end of prohibition signs.

Some Mathematical
Theorems Summarised

The Schröder–Bernstein Theorem:

If injective functions $f : A \rightarrow B$ and $g : B \rightarrow A$ between the sets A and B exist, then there exists a bijective function $h : A \rightarrow B$.

The Third Isomorphism Theorem:

Suppose that M and N are subgroups of group G and that M is a subgroup of N. Then M is normal in N, and there is an isomorphism from $(G/M) \,/\, (N/M)$ to G/N defined by $gM \cdot (N/M) \rightarrow gN$.

Kőnig's Bipartite Matching Theorem:

In a bipartite graph, the cardinality of a minimum cover is equal to the cardinality of a maximum matching.

Haken's Unknot Theorem:

It is decidable whether a given knot, represented by a knot diagram, is equivalent to the unknot.

The Lagrange Property for Moufang Loops:

If N is a finite Moufang loop then N has the Lagrange Property, which is to say that the order of any sub-loop divides the order of N.

Hilbert's Nullstellensatz ('The Theorem of Zeros'):

If k is a field and K is an algebraically closed field extension we have the polynomial ring $k[X_a, X_b \ldots X_n]$. Let J be an ideal in this ring. The algebraic set $V(J)$ defined by this ideal consists of all n-tuples $x = (x_a, x_b \ldots x_n)$ in K^n such that $f(x) = 0$ for all f in J. If p is some polynomial in $k[X_1, X_2 \ldots X_n]$ that vanishes on the algebraic set $V(J)$. This means that $p(x) = 0$ for all x in $V(J)$, and there exists a natural number r such that p^r is in J. (See also Zariski's Lemma.)

The Brouwer Fixed Point Theorem:

Every continuous function from the closed unit ball A^m to itself has at least one fixed point. (Where n is a positive integer, and the closed unit ball A^m is the set of all points in Euclidean n-space R^n which are no more than 1 from the origin.)

The Artin–Tate Lemma:

If C is Noetherian and R is a subalgebra of a commutative algebra S (where S is finitely generated as an R-module) then R is affine if S is affine.

The Fundamental Theorem of Galois Theory:

Given a field extension D/E that is Galois and finite, there is a one-to-one correspondence between the intermediate fields of this field extension and subgroups of the Galois group of this field extension.

Zariski's Lemma

If K is a field and K is also a finitely generated algebra over the field k then K is a finite field extension of k. It is important to note that Zariski's lemma is a proof of the weak form of Hilbert's Nullstellensatz (see above).

The Heine–Borel Theorem

This is a theory regarding the topology of metric spaces. For a subset S of Euclidean space R^n, these two statements are equivalent:

S is closed and bounded

S is compact, which means that every open cover of S has a finite subcover. This is the defining property of compact sets, called the Heine–Borel property.

Duck Identification

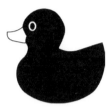

Melanitta americana
(BLACK SCOTER)

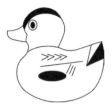

Anas discors
(BLUE-WINGED TEAL)

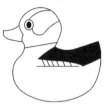

Bucephala albeola
(BUFFLEHEAD)

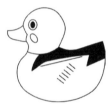

Bucephala clangula
(COMMON GOLDENEYE)

Mergus merganser
(COMMON MERGANSER)

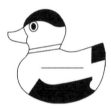

Somateria mollissima
(EIDER)

Tadorna tadorna
(COMMON SHELDUCK)

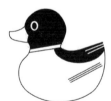

Mergus merganser
(GOOSEANDER)

Aythya collaris
(RING NECKED)

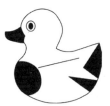

Aythya valisineria
(CANVASBACK)

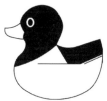

Aythya marila
(GREATER SCAUPE)

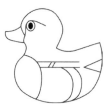

Anas clypeata
(NORTHERN
SHOVELLER)

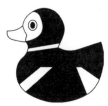

*Histrionicus
histrionicus*
(HARLEQUIN)

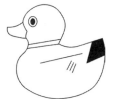

Anas platyrhynchos
(MALLARD)

Anas acuta
(NORTHERN PINTAIL)

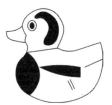

Clangula hyemalis
(OLD SQUAW)

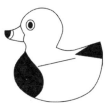

Aythya americana
(REDHEAD DUCK)

Aix sponsa
(WOOD DUCK)

How Sea Glass Is Made

Sea glass is glass that has physically and chemically weathered in the sea. It is most often found on beaches. One chemical element that contributes to its production is the salt in salt water. As a result of this and other weathering processes the glass becomes naturally frosted in the water. For sea glass to attain its characteristic texture and shape it takes perhaps 30, 40 or 50 years. It can even take as long as a hundred years.

In the water, small pieces of broken glass with sharp edges are tumbled and ground over a period of many years until the jagged edges becomes increasingly smoothed. The glass also loses its shine and becomes increasingly opaque as part of the same process. The glass may originate as pieces of glass from broken bottles; it can also come from jars, plates, windows, windshields, ceramics or even shipwrecks. Sea glass can be found off coasts all over the world, including: Argentina, Australia, Bermuda, Canada, China, Dominican Republic, France, Hawaii, India, Italy, Mexico, Puerto Rico, Scotland, Spain, Sri Lanka and the Continental United States.

The optimal time for finding sea glass is during perigean and proxigean spring tides, and during the first low tide after a storm. (Perigean tides happen three or four times a year when the perigee of the Moon coincides with a spring tide, which is when the Earth, Sun and Moon are most closely aligned, every two weeks or so; while a proxigean tide is an abnormally high tide that happens when the Moon is at its closest point to the Earth in the new Moon or full Moon phase.)

The colour of sea glass is determined by its source. The most common colours of sea glass are green, brown and white (clear). Less common colours include jade, amber (which usually originates in old bottles for medicine, spirits, whisky and early bleach bottles), golden amber (mostly used for spirit bottles), a particular shade of lime green (from old soft drink bottles), a deeper green and soft blue (usually from soft drink bottles, medicine bottles, ink bottles and fruit jars).

Less common colours of sea glass include a specific shade of green that was used in early twentieth-century fizzy drink and beer bottles. Purple sea glass is rare, as is yellow, cloudy white (from milk glass), cobalt blue, cornflower blue and aqua blue. The rarest colours are grey, pink, teal, black, yellow, turquoise, red and orange. Black glass sometimes has its origins in sturdy eighteenth-century gin, beer and wine bottles. Black glass can sometimes appear green or brown when you hold it up to the light. Gas bubbles trapped in old glass, and other kinds of impurities and irregularities, were more common in early glass production and can thus be used as an additional way of identifying possible sources and dates for the origin of a particular piece of sea glass. Early hand-blown bottles have more flaws, whereas those made in a mould have fewer flaws. Older bottles had thicker glass also, which means they can produce larger individual pieces of sea glass.

Particular substances are thus associated with particular colours and shapes of bottles, and the same can be said of the country of origin of the original glass. Medicines and alcoholic drinks were frequently sold in green bottles. Olive green was often used for gin, but brown was also used, as well as certain shades of blue. Whisky was often packaged in green and brown bottles. The alcohol bottles for substances being transported by sea were often square, as this is the shape that is most efficient when it comes to packing a quantity of bottles into a square or rectangular crate. Poisons were generally sold in blue bottles. Early trading ports are good places to find early examples of sea glass. In Jamaica, for instance, it is sometimes possible to find Spanish, African, English, American, Indian and Chinese glass, but the majority of black glass found on the island of Jamaica is English glass produced from the seventeenth to nineteenth centuries.

Staring Contest with 48 Cats

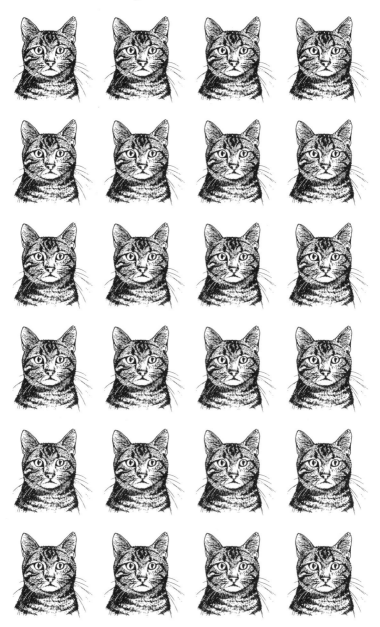

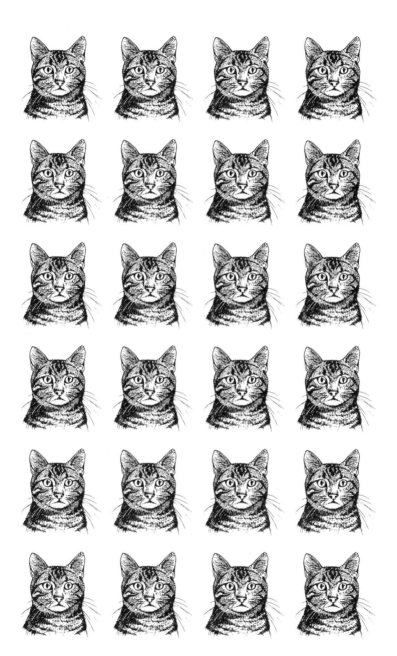

Counting Grains of Sand

In *The Sand Reckoner* the ancient Greek philosopher Archimedes attempted to find a way to count how many grains of sand it would take to fill up the universe. Imagine the number of grains of sand on a beach. This would be a very large number, although not infinite. Then imagine the number of grains of sand on another beach. If you add the two together, you have a number bigger than either of the numbers you started with.

Now imagine that the ocean between the two beaches is empty and, instead of being filled with water, it is filled with sand. Then imagine that all of the beaches and all of the oceans on the planet are filled with sand. How could we count so many individual grains of sand? Now imagine that every planet in the solar system has been turned to sand, and all the gaps in between all of the planets have been filled with sand. That would be a lot of sand.

Next, imagine that it is not just this solar system that has been filled with sand, but every star system, every galaxy – even the black holes have been filled with sand. That is how many grains of sand we would need to count in order to count how many grains of sand would be needed to fill the universe with sand.

Archimedes started with the myriad (10,000), the largest number the Greeks had a symbol for. This is probably barely enough to count the grains of sand on one beach, but it is a start. Next, he imagined a myriad of myriads (100,000,000). He took this as the unit in a second order of numbering. Then for the third order of numbering he imagined 100,000,000 multiplied by itself 100,000,000 times, which would be a myriad of myriads multiplied by itself a myriad of a myriad times.

His numbering system continued up to the fourth order, the unit for which was a myriad of a myriad of a myriad multiplied by itself a myriad of a myriad of a myriad times and then again by a myriad of a myriad of a myriad times. For his fourth order the unit was a myriad of a myriad of a myriad of a myriad times multiplied by itself a myriad of a myriad of a myriad of a myriad times and then again by a myriad of a myriad of a myriad of a myriad times and finally one more time a myriad of a myriad of a myriad of a myriad times.

By Archimedes's calculations this was quite a large number, possibly big enough to count how many grains of sand there would be if the Earth was made entirely of sand. However, to fill the universe with sand he needed larger numbers. So for the fifth order of numbers the unit was a myriad of a myriad of a myriad of a myriad of a myriad times multiplied by itself a myriad of a myriad of a myriad of a myriad of a myriad times and then again by a myriad of a myriad of a myriad of a myriad of a myriad times and then again by a myriad of a myriad of a myriad of a myriad of a myriad times and finally one more time a myriad of a myriad of a myriad of a myriad of a myriad of times.

This gave Archimedes numbers large enough to possibly fill the solar system with sand. But he still had a distance to go to entirely fill the universe with sand. For the sixth order the unit was a myriad of a myriad of a myriad of a myriad of a myriad of a myriad times multiplied by itself a myriad of a myriad of a myriad of a myriad of a myriad times and then again by a myriad of a myriad of a myriad of a myriad of a myriad of a myriad times and then again by a myriad of a myriad of a myriad of a myriad of a myriad of a myriad times and then again by a myriad of a myriad of a myriad of a myriad of a myriad of a myriad times and finally one more time a myriad of a myriad of a myriad of a myriad of a myriad of times.

For the seventh order of numbers, which was needed to get closer towards the extremely large numbers that Archimedes required, the unit was a myriad of a myriad of a myriad of a myriad of a myriad of a myriad of a myriad times multiplied by itself a myriad of a myriad of a myriad of a myriad of a myriad of a myriad of a myriad.

Visualisation:
Knitting a Cardigan[1]

Imagine you are knitting. With a reasonably large needle, start by slowly and carefully casting on 74 stitches. Then cast on 47 stitches for the right sleeve, and knit to the end of the row. Purl one row, and bind off. You should have 121 stitches at the end of this row. Next cast on 47 stitches for the left sleeve. Knit one, then purl one, then knit one, then purl one, and so on until the end of the row, at which point you should have 168 stitches.

Carefully bind off with three stitches then keep knitting across the row. Now move on to the second row, and gradually work in the textured stitch until the piece measures about 7 inches. About 17 inches from the cast you will, of course, need to make stitches for sleeves. Knit 68 stitches and stitch one stitch to a stitch holder for the right shoulder, then bind off the 27 stitches at the centre, before knitting to the end of the row for the left shoulder.

Continue in textured stitch until the sleeve measures 17 inches from the stitches you already cast on for the sleeve then end the process with a right-side row. Bind off with 49 stitches for the left sleeve, and continue in textured stitch. About 27 stitches should be left at the end of the process. Carefully continue in textured stitch until the left front measures 14 inches.

Now you need to carefully bind off with three stitches then keep knitting across the row. Again you should be using the knit one, purl one, knit one, purl one technique. You will end up with 58 stitches remaining on the needle. Slowly, patiently, work in the textured stitch. Purl one row, and bind off. Bind off with two stitches then knit across – this will give you about 62 stitches and should take several minutes of careful knitting.

1 Disclaimer: The authors take no responsibility for the resulting cardigan.

Now, carefully bind off with four stitches, and continue in textured stitch – 65 stitches should remain. Knit and purl for about three minutes. Bind off the resulting stitches, then continue with a different size of needle, either larger or smaller than the last needle, and continue in textured stitch – 62 stitches should remain.

From the bound-off stitches for the sleeve, continue with a careful right-side row, then purl a row and bind off. Stitch 142 stitches around the right shoulder from the stitch holder. Now we need a larger needle, so you can work a wrong side row. Rejoin the yarn, of course, before continuing with this process.

Bind off with 48 stitches, knit to the end of the row – 19 stitches should remain for the left front. Continue in textured stitch as established until the right front and the left front look vaguely similar to one another then end with a right-side row. Purl one row, and bind off. To make the stitches even across an edge use markers to divide the edge in thirds.

From one side, with a smaller needle, knit 56 stitches evenly spaced across the wrist edge of either sleeve. Carefully bind off with 3 stitches then keep knitting across the row. Rib for 8 inches or 5 minutes, whichever is shorter.

Continue in textured stitch until the right sleeve looks similar to the left sleeve, then knit another row. Bind off. Purl three stitches to the left then three stitches to the right. Repeat for both sleeves and the collar. Fold the cardigan and sew the side and sleeve seams, as well as the cuffs. The right and left halves should look similar. From the side, with a larger needle, knit 123 stitches spaced across the right front edge, from the edge up to the centre.

Work in stitches until the collar measures 9 or 10 inches. Bind off, and purl one, then knit one, then purl one. Find a smaller needle, then knit one, and purl one, and then repeat from the start.

What Time Is It?

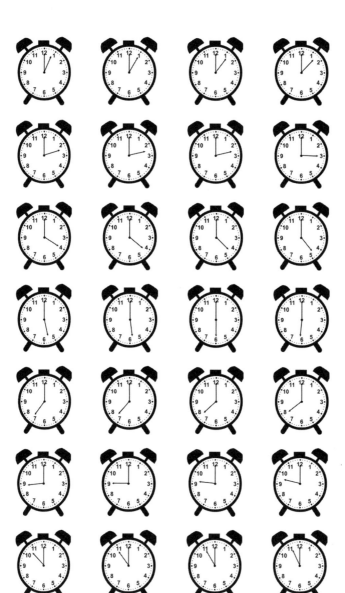

The Story of the Lithuanian Monarchy

The state of Lithuania was formed in the 1230s. At the time there were dual threats from the Teutonic Knights in the west and the Livonian Order in the north. The Livonian Order was an order of military monks established by the third Bishop of Riga in 1202. They would eventually merge with the Teutonic Order (another military order founded in the late twelfth century in Acre) following a defeat by the Samogitians and Semigallians at the Battle of Schaulen (also known as Saule). Following this battle there were further revolts against the military orders among groups such as the Curonians, Selonians and Oeselians. These were a variety of ethic and tribal groups in the Baltic region. The Curonians lived on the coast of the Baltic Sea in what would now be known as western Latvia or Lithuania and gave their name to the modern region of Courland. Their modern descendants include the Kuršininkai of the Curonian Spit. The Selonians lived in what would now be known as southeastern Latvia or northeastern Lithuania. Little is known about them, although their burial traditions show a similarity to the Latgalians, who were an eastern Baltic tribe who lived in the eastern part of present day Vidzeme. The Samogitians lived in the western part of modern Lithuania, and were closely related to the Semigallians and Curonians. The Semigallians lived somewhat to the east of the Samogitians, in south central Lithuania and northern Latvia.

In the 1230s some but not all of these ethnic and tribal groups came together into the state of Lithuania. The first ruler was Mindaugas, who was the grand duke, and who also became king in 1253 following his conversion to Christianity, which allowed him to form an alliance with the Livonians. However, in 1261 his alliance with the Livonians collapsed, and he was eventually assassinated by his relatives Treniota and Duke Daumantas.

Most of what we know about Mindaugas comes from two contemporary documents, *The Livonian Rhymed Chronicle* and

The Hypatian Codex. The Livonian Rhymed Chronicle is a historical chronicle of events written in High German, in rhyme. *The Hypatian Codex* is itself made up of three separate documents in the Old Church Slavonic language, *The Primary Chronicle, The Kiev Chronicle* and *The Galician–Volhynian Chronicle. The Primary Chronicle* is a historical chronicle that originated in the Kiev area. *The Kiev Chronicle* is also presumed to be related to the Kiev area. And *The Galician–Volhynian Chronicle* is a historical document relating to the Principality of Galicia–Volhynia, which is not far from Kiev.

The subsequent rulers of Lithuania should technically be referred to as grand dukes rather than as kings, although they all referred to themselves as kings. Treniota followed Mindaugas to the throne but was himself assassinated in 1265. The son of Mindaugas, Vaišvilkas, was the next ruler, but he abdicated in favour of his brother-in-law Švarnas, who was the only ruler of the shortlived House of Monomakhovichi. The next two leaders were Traidenis and Daumantas, who expanded the territory of Lithuania further into the territories of the Sudovians, Semigallians and Black Ruthenians. The Sudovians (also known as the Yotvingians, Suduvians, Jatvians or Jatvingians) lived in parts of modern Poland, Belarus and Lithuania. Black Ruthenia was in the region of modern-day Navahrudak (or Novogrudok), on the upper reaches of the Neman River. Very little else is known about Daumantas as he is mentioned no more than once in *The Livonian Rhymed Chronicle, The Primary Chronicle, The Kiev Chronicle* or *The Galician–Volhynian Chronicle*.

Following the brief reign of Daumantas, Lithuania was ruled by the House of Gediminas. The grand dukes of this dynasty included Butigeidis, Butvydas, Vytenis, Gediminas himself, Jaunutis, Algirdas, Jogaila, Kęstutis, Jogaila (the second) and, of course, Vytautas the Great. Following Vytautas the Great there were numerous further grand dukes in the House of Gediminas.

Facts and Figures:
the Philately of Mauritius

- The first Mauritian postage stamps were issued in 1847.

- The image on the stamps was created by Joseph Osmond Barnard.

- People featured on Mauritian stamps include the missionary Pierre Poivre.

- The Poivre Islands coral atoll is also named after Pierre Poivre.

- One of the original stamps is known as the one penny red brown. It had a face value of one penny and was a reddish brownish colour.

- The other original 1847 stamp is known as the 'two pence blue'. It is blue and had a face value of two pennies.

- An envelope carrying both the two pence blue and the one penny red brown was sold in Zurich in 1993.

- Some of the original stamps were used on letters sent out by the wife of the governor of Mauritius.

- The first printing of the 1847 stamps included the words 'post office', but this was later changed to 'post paid'.

- The one pence stamp was used for post sent within a town, the two pence stamp was used for other purposes.

- The one pence and two pence rates were stipulated by Mauritius's Ordinance No. 13, which set out the postal rates that would be used.

- The one penny orange was issued in 1854. It is orange.

- The original engraving used on the stamp was later recreated by Jules Lapirot and subsequently by Robert Sherwin.

- The version with the engraving by Jules Lapirot is known as the 'Lapirot issue'.

- The version with the engraving by Robert Sherwin is known as the 'Sherwin issue'. It has been discovered that the Sherwin issue was printed in sheets of 12 stamps.

- Construction of the Mauritius Postal Museum commenced in 1865.

- The Mauritius Postal Museum was inaugurated and opened in 1868.

Mind Whirls: GPS Navigation

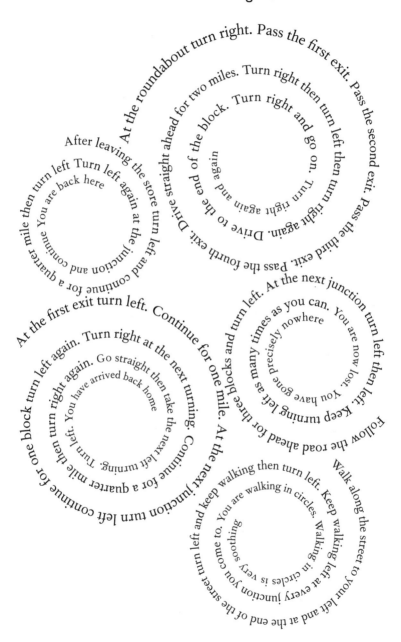

The Administration of the Mauryan
Empire in India's Golden Age

Chandragupta Maurya, who ruled from the Mauryan Empire, was advised by Kautilya, the author of the *Arthashastra* (*Science of Material Gain*). This laid out the foundations of a centralised but hierarchically distributed government, with a strong focus on important issues such as administration. As a whole, the empire was made up of provinces, districts and villages, each of which was run by local officials, who carried out the functions that were delegated to them by the central administration. The king was the head of the executive, and he appointed the subordinate officials, including ministers and other officers of the administration. The council of ministers (the *Mantri Parishad*) advised the king on his decisions and helped to delegate them down to more junior officials of the administration. The number of ministers in the council of ministers varied, depending on events. Not all ministers were required to attend all meetings. Beneath the council of ministers was the civil service of the Mauryan Empire, who carried out the central executive, judicial and revenue offices in a highly efficient manner. Each department within the civil service was run by a superintendent (*Adhyaksha*). Two other types of officials were the *Samaharta* (the collectors of revenue) and the *Sannidhata*, who was the officer in charge of the administrative functioning of the treasury.

The part of the kingdom that was directly ruled by the king was made up of numerous provinces (*Janapadas*). Some of the capitals of the provinces were Taxila, Ujjain, Tosali, Suvarnagiri and Pataliputra. Each province was made up of numerous districts and each district was subdivided into smaller sub-districts. Some of the sub-districts were further subdivided with the village being the smallest possible sub-district of a sub-district. The governor of each province dealt with the daily administrative tasks relating specifically to that province, in association with those parts of the central administration that related specifically to the province. The governor was also assisted in this task by district officers, reporters and clerks who were assigned to the particular province in question.

The Mauryan municipal administrative system added further complexities to the situation. There is, for instance, a historical account of the administrative operation of the municipal board of Pataliputra. This was overseen by a board, which had 30 members. The board was subdivided into six committees. Each committee was made up of five members. Sometimes these committees would split up into smaller subcommittees, depending on what the purpose of the committee was and the administrative task it was to undertake. Collectively the board and the committees ran the administration of the city. The main areas the committees oversaw were industry, citizens, registration, trade and commerce, manufacturing and the administrative collection of excise duties and custom duties.

There were numerous sources of revenue for the state, each of which required a range of specific administrative tasks. Land revenue was one important source of revenue. There were also duties on a variety of commodities and trades, for instance, forestry, water, mining and the creation of currency. The revenue was used to fund a variety of branches of the state, including the military, the officials, public projects, public construction and the administrative bureaucracy that undertook each of these tasks. These included excise duty, forest taxes, water taxes, mines and coinage. Much of the state revenue was used for paying the army or the officials of the royal government, or was spent on charities and on different public works like irrigation projects and road construction. In the reign of Ashoka, further reforms were applied, for instance, to the methods of administration, as well as to the executive, legislative and judicial branches of the administrative bureaucracy. There was also a new class of officers created: the *Dhamma Mahamatras*.

The World's Longest Tournament
Chess Game

The longest chess game ever played in a tournament took 269 moves between Ivan Nikolić and Goran Arsović, in Belgrade 1989. It lasted 20 hours and ended in a draw. If you want to recreate the extraordinary event, here is a brief account of the moves.

Nikolić started by moving a pawn to d4. Arsović responded by moving a knight to f6. Nikolić moved another pawn, this time to c4, while Arsović responded with a pawn to g6. Nikolić moved a knight to c3 and Arsović moved a bishop to g7.

For his fourth move Nikolić moved a third pawn, this time to e4. And Arsović responded with a pawn to d6. Then Nikolić moved a knight to f3. Excitingly, Arsović now castled. Nikolić moved a bishop to e2 and Arsović moved a knight to d7 from b.

On the seventh move Nikolić belatedly responded to Arsović castling by castling himself. Arsović moved a pawn to e5. Nikolić moved a castle (or rook) to e1 and Arsović moved a rook to e8. On the ninth move Nikolić moved a bishop to f1 and Arsović responded by moving a pawn to h6. Then Nikolić moved a pawn to d5 and Arsović moved a knight to h7. In response to this Nikolić moved a castle to b1, whereupon Arsović moved a pawn to f5.

The two players had now reached their twelfth and thirteenth moves, which involved pawns moving respectively to d2 and f4 and then to b4 and g5. Nikolić then turned to his knight, which he moved to b3, and Arsović moved a bishop to f8. Then Nikolić also moved a bishop to e2 and Arsović moved a knight from d to f6. Another two pawns were moved to c5 and g4.

At this point the game burst into life as the players exchanged pawns, Nikolić taking the pawn on d6 (from c) and Arsović responding by taking the same square with the pawn from c. Next Nikolić moved a pawn to a3, while Arsović responded with a knight moved to g5.

For his nineteenth move Nikolić moved his bishop to f1 while Arsović moved a castle to e7. Then came the first queen move of the game, with Nikolić deploying his queen out to d3, while Arsović responded with a castle to g7. Even more excitement was to follow as Nikolić moved his king to h1 and Arsović moved his queen to e8. At this point the game was in the balance.

Nikolić moved his knight to d2, while Arsović played for time by moving a pawn to g3. On the twenty-third move Nikolić took the piece on g3 and once again Arsović responded by taking back (with the aggressors in each case coming from f). Then another capture followed, with Nikolić's queen taking the piece on g3. Arsović couldn't immediately respond with another capture so instead moved his knight to h3.

As the tension in the room continued to rise the two men both moved their queens, respectively to f3 and g6. Then Nikolić moved a pawn to c4 and Arsović responded with a knight to d7. Nikolić moved a bishop to d3 and Arsović moved a knight to g5. The next move was the twenty-eighth move for each player, a bishop to g5 for Nikolić, followed by Arsović belatedly evening up the capture count by taking that piece with his queen. Then Nikolić moved his knight to e3 while Arsović responded with a castle to e8.

Pressing on with his knight strategy, Nikolić moved onto e2, whereas Arsović preferred his bishop, which he moved to e7. Next, both players moved their castles, Nikolić from b to d1 and Arsović to f8. Next, both players deployed their knight, Nikolić to f5 and Arsović to g4. The game was growing increasingly exciting with every move, although it is clear that both players were being somewhat defensive in their mindset.

Next, Nikolić moved the knight from e to g3 and Arsović moved a pawn to h5. We had now reached the thirty-fourth move: Nikolić took his king to g1, while Arsović advanced the same pawn by another square to h4. Then the players exchanged pieces as each moved on to g4 and the game continued.

The Habsburg Empire:
the Early Years

The Habsburg Empire was named after Habsburg Castle (also known as Habichtsburg) overlooking the Aar River. The castle was built in 1020 by Count Radbot and his brother-in-law Werner. Radbot's son became the first Count of Habsburg. He was the grandfather of Albert III, who was Count of Zurich and the landgrave of Upper Alsace. (A landgrave was a count with jurisdiction over a particular territory.) After the death of Albert III and of Rudolf II of Habsburg the associated territories were divided between Albert IV and Rudolf III; however, the descendants of Rudolf III sold their territory back to the descendants of Albert IV. It was his son Rudolf IV who became German king in 1273, although this meant that rather than being known as Rudolf IV he became known as Rudolf I. His sons Albert (who would become Albert I) and Rudolf (Rudolf II of Austria) inherited land including most of Austria as their territory.

Rudolf II renounced his share in the territories but, after the death of Albert I, there were problems with how the territory should be divided. The problems were eventually settled, with Rudolf IV taking the senior position in a partition of the territory with his brothers Albert III and Leopold III.

By this time Rudolf III was ruling Austria and Frederick I had become King of Germany (as Frederick III) while Albert V of Austria became German king (as Albert II). His son Ladislaus Posthumus also inherited the crown of Hungary in 1446. He was the last male descendant of Albert III. At this point the line of descent from Leopold III had divided into two surviving branches, the Inner Austrian branch and the Tyrolean branch. Frederick V was the senior member of the former and he now became the German king, though he was known as Frederick III rather than Frederick V.

One of the Frederick's first acts was to ratify the Habsburgs' use of the title of 'Archduke of Austria' (which had earlier been arrogated for or to them by Rudolf IV). His son Maximilian united the Austrian hereditary lands when Sigismund of Tyrol abdicated in his favour (in 1490).

Maximilian married Mary, the heiress of Burgundy, which meant that their son Philip would inherit the territories of Charles the Bold, including Artois, the Netherlands, Luxembourg and the County of Burgundy or Franche-Comté. Philip went on to marry Joan, heiress of Castile and Aragon as well as other places such as Naples, Sicily and Sardinia. Maximilian was succeeded in the role of Habsburg monarch by Charles V.

It is important to be precise about how we talk about the Habsburgs as there are various different nomenclatures that can be applied to the dynasty. The Habsburg Monarchy (*Habsburgermonarchie*) is essentially a way of referring to monarchy that had a descendant of the Habsburgs as its titular head. This is contrasted with the Habsburg Empire (*Habsburgerreich*) which is the empire ruled over by the descendants of the Habsburgs.

The core part of the Habsburg dynasty's territory that was ruled over directly by the Habsburg monarchy was known as either the Habsburg Hereditary Lands or Austrian Hereditary Lands (*Habsburgische Erblande* or *Österreichische Erblande*). These are to be contrasted with the Austrian Monarchy (*Österreichische Monarchie*) and also with other monarchically ruled areas. In later centuries other pieces of nomenclature were used. For instance, the Austrian Empire (*Kaisertum Österreich*) could refer to the empire ruled from Austria or to a 'widespreading domain' thereof. Austria–Hungary would become the official name of the monarchy's territory – this was also sometimes referred to as the Double Monarchy (*Doppel-Monarchie*) or, colloquially, as the Danubian Monarchy (*Donaumonarchie*).

Interesting Facts about Oak Trees

- *Quercus canariensis* is better known by its colloquial name, Algerian oak.

- Blue oak (*Quercus douglasii*) can also be known as iron oak.

- Galls that affect oak species include oak artichoke gall, oak marble gall, oak apple gall, knopper gall and spangle gall.

- Ring-cupped oaks (*Cyclobalanopsis*) are distinguished from the *Quercus* subgenus by the concrescent rings of scales on their acorns.

- Bur oak (*Quercus macrocarpa*) is sometimes misspelled as burr oak.

- The wood of an oak has a density of about 0.75g/cm^3.

- Californian oak (*Quercus kelloggii*) is a native species of California.

- *Quercus chrysolepis* (canyon live oak) sometimes grows in canyons.

- Champion oak (*Quercus rubra*) is sometimes known as northern red oak.

- Eastern black oak (*Quercus velutina*) can also be called yellow oak. It has blackish outer bark but its inner bark is yellow.

- The coat of arms of Eigersund in Norway features an oak leaf.

- Island oak (*Quercus tomentella*) can be grown on islands.

- Mossycup white oak (*Quercus macrocarpa*) is another name for bur oak (see above).

- Dyer's oak is another name for eastern black oak (see above).

- *Quercus robur* can be known as common oak, pedunculate oak, European oak or English oak.

- *Quercus velutina* (commonly known as eastern black oak or yellow oak, see above) can also be called yellowbark oak or spotted oak.

- Within the genus *Quercus*, the section *Mesobalanus* is sometimes included in the section *Quercus.*

- Oaks grow very, very slowly, although some species grow faster than others.

- There are over 600 species of oak, although some of them are very similar to each other.

A CATALOGUE OF SPOONS

Absinthe spoon
Bar spoon
Berry spoon
Bouillon spoon
Caddy spoon
Cappuccino spoon
Caviar spoon
Cheese spoon
Chinese spoon
Chowder spoon
Coffee spoon
Cream spoon
Cream-soup spoon
Custard spoon
Cutty
Demitasse spoon
Dessert spoon
Ear spoon
Egg spoon
French-sauce spoon
Fruit spoon
Grapefruit spoon or
    orange spoon
Gumbo spoon
Horn spoon
Ice-cream fork
Iced-tea spoon
Jelly or jam spoon
Ladle

Long drink spoon
Marrow spoon
Melon spoon
Mocha spoon
Mote spoon
Mustard spoon
Olive spoon
Parfait spoon
Plastic spoon
Rice spoon
Salad spoon
Salt spoon
Saucier spoon
Serving spoon
Silver spoon
Slotted spoon
Soup spoon
Spaghetti spoon
Spork
Stirrer
Sugar spoon
Sugar tongs
Table spoon
Tablespoon
Tea spoon
Teaspoon
Treacle spoon
Wooden spoon
Yoghurt spoon

Notable Events of the Thirteenth Century

1200 The Peace of Goulet
1201 Birth of King Thibault IV of Navarre
1202 The trial of the Duke of Burgundy in France
1203 Muhammad of Ghor conquers part of India
1204 Greek kingdom of Epirus established
1205 Death of Ladislaus III of Hungary
1206 The Livonian Brothers of the Sword and the
    Semigallians conquer Livs
1207 Death of Reinmar the Old of Hagenau
1208 Sverker the Younger deposed as King of Sweden
1209 Otto IV crowned Emperor in Rome
1210 Otto IV excommunicated by Pope Innocent III
1211 Birth of Ibn Khallikan, Kurdish scholar
1212 Work commences on Rheims cathedral (and continues
    for 99 years)
1213 The Council of St Albans meets in England
1214 Sinope, a city on the Black Sea, conquered by the
    Seljuq Turks
1215 Birth of Hartmann von der Aue, German poet
1216 Mstislav the Daring and Konstantin of Rostov win the
    battle of Lipitsa
1217 Mukhali made chief of operations in North China by
    Genghis Khan
1218 Adoption of the Dannebrog as national flag of
    Denmark
1219 King Valdemar II of Denmark conquers Tallinn in the
    Battle of Lyndanisse
1220 Boys' choir founded at the Kreuz-Kirche in Dresden
1221 Abdication of Emperor Juntoku
1222 Death of Alexios Megas Komnenos, Emperor of
    Trebizond
1223 Sancho II crowned King of Portugal

Count the Sheep Again

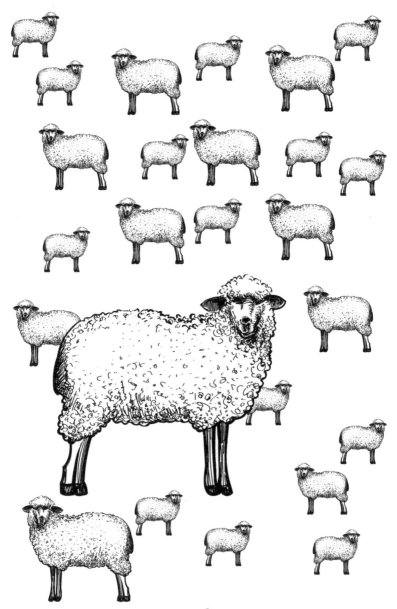

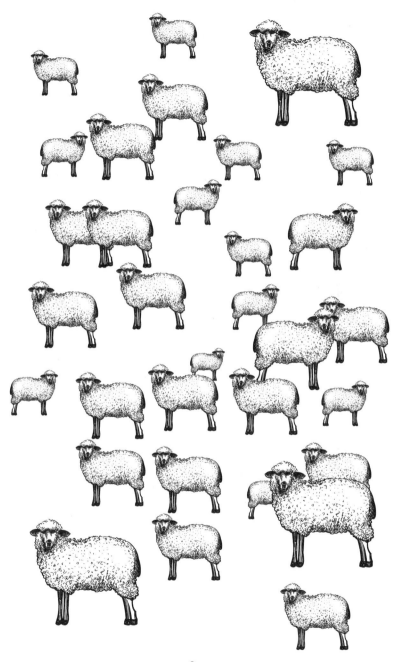

A Precise Chronology of the
Devonian Period

When we talk about the Devonian Period as though it were a single period in time there is an immediate and grave danger of imprecision. The entire period lasted for approximately 60 million years from 419.2 million years ago to 358.9 million years ago[1] (so to be slightly more precise 60.3 million years in total[2]), and thus we need to be cautious about mis-describing any of its subdivisions or indeed the faunal stages of the subdivisions.

Firstly, we need to divide the Devonian Period into three subdivisions: the Early Devonian Period, the Middle Devonian Period and the Late Devonian Period. The Early Devonian Period lasted from 419.2 million years ago to 393.3 million years ago, so lasted for 25.9 million years. The Middle Devonian Period lasted from 393.3 million years ago to 382.7 million years ago, so lasted for 10.6 million years. The Late Devonian Period lasted from 382.7 million years ago to 358.9 million years ago, so lasted for 23.8 million years.

Next, we need to subdivide each of these periods into shorter faunal stages. The Early Devonian Period commenced with the Lochkovian stage. This lasted from 419.2 million years ago to 410.8 million years ago, 8.4 million years in total. An example of a species from this period is the Agnathan of the Drepanaspis taxa.

The Lochkovian stage was followed by the Pragian stage. This lasted until 407.6 million years ago, and thus lasted about 3.2 million years. An important lagerstätte (a sedimentary deposit with

---

1 All dates given are those ratified by the International Commission on Stratigraphy and are correct at the date of writing.

2 Although it should be noted that all dates given here have the possibility of being incorrect by up to 3 million years. So while this chronology is precise as to the dates currently ratified by the ICS, those dates are inherently imprecise and subject to future revision.

well-preserved fossil evidence) of the Pragian stage is the Rhynie chert, as found in Scottish sedimentary deposits.

The third and final faunal stage of the Early Devonian Period is the Emsian stage. This lasted from 407.6 million years ago to 393.3 million years ago, so it lasted about 14.3 million years. An example of a species found in this period is the placoderm of the taxa *Gemuendina* found at Hunsrück Slate Formation in Germany.

The Middle Devonian Period only has two faunal stages as opposed to the three faunal stages of the Early Devonian Period. The first faunal stage was the Eifelian stage, which lasted from 393.3 million years ago to 387.7 million years ago, which means that it lasted for about 5.6 million years. It is named after the Eifel Hills in western Germany where the GSSP is visible in the Wetteldorf Richtschnitt. (A GSSP is an internationally agreed reference point on a stratigraphic section that can be used to define the lower boundary of a geological time-scale stage.) An example of a species from the Eifelian stage is an arthropod of the taxa *Jaekelopterus*.

The second and final faunal stage of the Middle Devonian Period is the Givetian stage, which lasted from 387.7 million years ago to 382.7 million years ago, meaning that it lasted for 5 million years. A typical species of the period is a tetrapodomorph of the taxa *Elpistostege*. This is a vertebrate resembling a tetrapod, which would go extinct in the first faunal stage of the Late Devonian Period.

Like the Middle Devonian Period, the Late Devonian Period was divided into just two faunal stages (meaning that there were seven faunal stages in the entirety of the Devonian Period). The first faunal stage of the Late Devonian Period was the Frasnian stage, which lasted from 382.7 million years ago to 372.2 million years ago, meaning that it lasted for 10.5 million years. An interesting species of the Frasnian stage was an amphibian of the *Obruchevichthys* taxa, an extinct genus of tetrapod.

A Slow Train through Norway

Some of the Norwegian Broadcasting Corporation's finest moments have occurred in their forays into slow television. The groundbreaking programme in this genre was their *Bergensbanen – minutt for minutt* which showed the seven-hour journey by train from Bergen to Oslo in live time. As well as showing every minute of the journey, this included showing the train stopping at some of the stations on the line, which include Arna, Dale, Voss, Mjølfjell, Upsete, Myrdal, Hallingskeid, Finse, Haugastøl, Ustaoset, Geilo, Ål, Gol, Nesbyen, Flå, Hønefoss, Vikersund, Hokksund, Drammen and Asker. (There are also numerous smaller stations in between the stations mentioned above.) The journey is 496 kilometres. The station at the highest altitude is Finse, at 1,222 metres. The viewers were also able to enjoy watching the train go through the following significant tunnels: Ulriken Tunnel (7,670 metres) before Arna station, Arnanipa Tunnel (2,190 metres) between Arna and Tunestveit Junction, Takvam Tunnel (251 metres) and Tunestveidt Tunnel (61 metres), which are between Tunestveidt Junction and Takvam station, which is four stops before Stanghelle station, with the intervening stations being Trengereid, Bogegrend and Vaksdal stations, Bolstad Tunnel (110 metres) and Trollkona Tunnel (8,043 metres), which are between Stanghelle station and Bolstadøyri station, Røvstona Tunnel (542 metres), which is between Bolstadøyri station and Jørnevik station, and finally the Hærnes Tunnel (3,336 metres), Kattegjelet Tunnel (529 metres), Kattegjel Viaduct Tunnel (19 metres) and Lillevik Tunnel (292 metres) (all of which are between Jørnevik station and Evanger station, which are before Mjølfjell on the journey from Bergen to Oslo). There are 182 tunnels in total on the journey, so we have only mentioned the most notable ones in this brief summary. Thereafter the journey continues over the Hardangervidda plateau with fewer significant tunnels, although the train does pass over the Svenkerud Bridge over the river Hallingdalselva between Gol and Nesbyen stations.

In 2010 the Norwegian Broadcasting Corporation showed a shorter 28-minute film *Bybanen i Bergen – minutt for minutt*, which showed the shorter trip on the Bergen Light Rail from Nesttun to Bergen. This showed the journey minute by minute as well as the stops at the various stations en route. This would have included some of the following stations: Nesttun, Nesttun senter, Skjoldskiftet, Mårdalen, Skjold, Lagunen, Folldalstunnelen, Råstølen, Sandslivegen, Sandslimarka, Kokstad, Birkelandsskiftet terminal, Kokstadflaten, Kokstad depot and Bergen lufthavn Flesland.

It is relevant to note that this line has since been extended and one could now make the continuous journey from Byparken through the stations and tunnels at Nonneseteren, Bystasjonen, Nygård, Florida, Nygård Bridge, Danmarksplass, Kronstad, Brann stadion, Wergeland, Wergeland Tunnel, Sletten, Slettebakken, Slettebakken Tunnel, Fantoft, Fantoft Tunnel, Paradis, Tveiterås Tunnel, Hop and Nesttun (and from there onwards via the same stations that we have already mentioned).

Also in 2010, the Norwegian Broadcasting Corporation showed *Flåmsbana – minutt for minutt*. This was a 58-minute-long depiction of the journey on the Flåm line, a 20.2-kilometre line that travels 863 metres (2,831 feet) from Myrdal to Flåm on the Sognefjord. We have noted that Myrdal is on the Bergen line. Starting from there, the Flåm line is a branch line. Starting from Myrdal the stations and tunnels are Toppen øvre Tunnel (101 metres), Toppen nedre Tunnel (80 metres), Vatnahalsen, Reinunga, Vatnahalsen Tunnel (889 metres), Bakli Tunnel (195 metres), Kjosfossen, Kjosfossen Tunnel (478 metres), Nåli Tunnel (1,341.5 metres) then Kårdal. After Kårdal comes Blomheller Tunnel (1,029 metres), which leads on to the station at Blomheller. Then there are four more tunnels between Blomheller and Berekvam: Melhus (178 metres), Melhusgjelet Tunnel (11 metres), Reppa Tunnel (133 metres) and Sjølskott Tunnel (39 metres).

Motorway Mindfulness

There is a large expanse of grey concrete in front of you. Look at the lines painted on it. It separates the road into three lanes. Concentrate on the lane you are driving along. A large red lorry is coming up behind you. It moves to the right-hand lane and passes you. In front of you are many cars all going in the same direction. This is a long road. There is no way you can turn off it for several miles. You just have to keep driving in a straight line. Concentrate on driving straight ahead. You cannot stop or turn around. This is your only available choice. You have to keep moving forwards in the same direction. To your left is a grassy bank, which is occasionally dotted with unusually small trees held up by wooden poles. This is all you can see. To your right is a barrier, and beyond that is an identical road with cars all travelling in the opposite direction. You must stay away from this road, but there is no turning back now. Ahead of you is a concrete bridge. It is grey and you cannot see the road that it is connected to on either side. To your left is the same high grassy bank; to your right is another high grassy bank. You have no idea what lies beyond: the grassy banks are designed to stop you from being distracted by the outside world. You just have to concentrate on the road ahead. For now there is nothing else to see. A blue car goes past very quickly on your right. Coming up on your left is a road from the outside world that allows other cars to join you, so you will be travelling together along this expanse of concrete. A white van is joining you and the other cars. You must move into the lane to your right to let them join in. Signs flash by telling you how many miles until you can leave this road. It is always too many. There are signs with the names of places you've never been and probably never will. Many are places you have never heard of. Who lives there? What is it like? Don't allow these thoughts to intrude.

Pickled Cucumbers: a World Almanac

- A pickled cucumber is a cucumber that has been pickled in brine, vinegar or another substance, or else left to sour through lacto-fermentation.

- In the USA and Canada a pickled cucumber can be referred to simply as a 'pickle'.

- The word 'pickle' in the UK does not generally refer to a pickled cucumber.

- Gherkins are traditionally burr gherkins (*Cucumis anguria*), which have a smaller fruit than the garden cucumber (*Cucumis sativus*).

- In fermented or crock pickles, either vinegar is added or the vegetables are fermented in salt brine over several weeks.

- Fresh or quick pickles are not fermented, but involve a quicker process by which vinegar and salt brine are poured onto the vegetables.

- Refrigerated and frozen pickles are prepared using standard processes

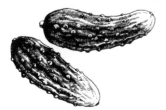

as above, but then they are stored in refrigerators or freezers.

- The Polish for a pickled cucumber is *ogórek kiszony/ogóriki kwaszone'* or *ogórek konserwowy*.

- A cucumber that has been pickled in brine is called a 'brine pickle'.

- Cucumbers that have been pickled with added sugar are called 'sweet pickles'.

- Some historians suggest that the first pickled cucumber dates to 2400 BC, but other historians have suggested a date of 2050 BC. Or, depending on how you translate the words in ancient documents, they may date back as far as 4000 BC.

- A cucumber that has been pickled in dill-flavoured vinegar is called a 'dill pickle'.

- Kosher dill pickles are not necessarily kosher.

- Pickled cucumbers flavoured with tarragon are known as *cornichons* in France.

- German pickles are called *Spreewald gherkins*. Hungarian pickles are called *savanyú uborka* or *kovászos uborka*.

'The Measure of Fidget'
by Francis Galton[1]

Latterly – no matter where – I was present at a crowded and expectant meeting. The communication proved tedious and I could not hear much of it, so from my position at the back of the platform I studied the expressions and gestures of the bored audience.

The feature that an instantaneous photograph, taken at any moment, would most prominently have displayed was the unequal horizontal interspace between head and head. When the audience is intent each person forgets his muscular weariness and skin discomfort, and he holds himself rigidly in the best position for seeing and hearing. As this is practically identical for persons who sit side by side, their bodies are parallel and again, as they are at much the same distance apart, their heads are correspondingly equidistant. But when the audience is bored several individuals cease to forget themselves and they begin to pay much attention to the discomforts attendant on sitting long in the same position.

They sway from side to side, each in his own way, and the intervals between their faces, which lie at the free end of the radius formed by their bodies, with their seat as the centre of rotation, vary greatly. I endeavoured to give numerical expression for this variability of distance, but for the present have failed. I was, however, perfectly successful in respect to another sign of mutiny against constraint, inasmuch as I found myself able to estimate the frequency of the fidget with much precision.

It happened that the hall was semi-circularly disposed and that small columns under the gallery were convenient as points of reference. From where I sat, 50 persons were included in each sector of which my eye formed the apex and any adjacent pair of columns

1 Published in the 25 June 1885 edition of the scientific journal *Nature*.

the boundaries. I watched most of these sections in turn, some of them repeatedly, and counted the number of distinct movements among the persons they severally contained.

It was curiously uniform, and about 45 per minute. As the sectors were rather too long for the eye to surely cover at a glance, I undoubtedly missed some movements on every occasion. Partly on this account and partly for the convenience of using round numbers, I will accept 50 movements per minute among 50 persons, or an average of one movement per minute in each person, as nearly representing the true state of the case.

The audience was mostly elderly; the young would have been more mobile. Circumstances now and then occurred that roused the audience to temporary attention, and the effect was twofold. First, the frequency of fidget diminished rather more than half; second, the amplitude and period of each movement were notably reduced. The swayings of head, trunk and arms had before been wide and sluggish, and when rolling from side to side the individuals seemed to 'yaw'; that is to say, they lingered in extreme positions. Whenever they became intent this peculiarity disappeared, and they performed their fidgets smartly.

Let me suggest to observant philosophers when the meetings they attend may prove to be dull, to occupy themselves in estimating the frequency, amplitude and duration of the fidgets of their fellow sufferers. They must do so during periods both of intentness and of indifference so as to eliminate what may be styled 'natural fidget', and then I think they may acquire the new art of giving numerical expression to the amount of boredom expressed by the audience generally during the reading of any particular memoir.

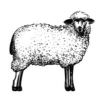

Chemical Reactions Revision

Synthesis reactions are those that can be described as A + B = AB.

$2\,Al\ (s) + 3\,Br_2\ (g) \rightarrow 2\,AlBr_3\ (s)$
$S_8\ (s) + 8\,O_2\ (g) \rightarrow 8\,SO_2\ (g)$
$2\,CO\ (g) + O_2\ (g) \rightarrow 2\,CO_2\ (g)$
$CaO\ (s) + CO_2\ (g) \rightarrow CaCO_3\ (s)$

By contrast decomposition reactions can be described as AB $\rightarrow$ A + B.

$2\,HgO\ (s) \rightarrow 2\,Hg\ (l) + O_2\ (g)$
$2\,N_2O_5\ (g) \rightarrow O_2\ (g) + 4\,NO_2\ (g)$
$2\,Cu(NO_3)\ 2\ (s) \rightarrow 2\,CuO\ (s) + 4\,NO_2\ (g) + O_2\ (g)$
$Mg(NO_3)\ 2\ (s) \rightarrow Mg(NO_2)\ 2\ (s) + O_2\ (g)$
$2\,KBrO_3\ (s) \rightarrow 2\,KBr\ (s) + 3\,O_2\ (g)$
$CaCO_3\ (s) \rightarrow CaO\ (s) + CO_2\ (g)$
$2\,Fe(OH)_3\ (s) \rightarrow Fe_2O_3\ (s) + 3\,H_2O\ (g)$
$2\,NH_4NO_3\ (s) \rightarrow 2\,N_2\ (g) + 4\,H_2O\ (g) + O_2\ (g)$
$(NH_4)\ 2\,Cr_2O_7\ (s) \rightarrow Cr_2O_3\ (s) + 4\,H_2O\ (g) + N_2\ (g)$
$(CaSO_4) \cdot 2\,H_2O\ (s) \rightarrow CaSO_4\ (s) + 2\,H_2O\ (g)$
$(NH_4)\ 2\,SO_4\ (s) \rightarrow 2\,NH_3\ (g) + H_2SO_4\ (l)$

Single-displacement reactions are those where two particular elements are substituted for another element in a compound.

$Cu\ (s) + 2\,AgNO_3\ (aq) \rightarrow Cu(NO_3)\ 2\ (aq) + 2\,Ag\ (s)$
$2\,Al\ (s) + Fe_2O_3\ (s) \rightarrow Al_2O_3\ (s) + 2\,Fe\ (l)$
$Fe\ (s) + 2\,HCl\ (aq) \rightarrow FeCl_2\ (aq) + H_2\ (g)$

$$Ca\ (s) + 2H_2O\ (l) \rightarrow Ca(OH)_2\ (aq) + H_2\ (g)$$
$$Mg\ (s) + 2H_2O\ (g) \rightarrow Mg(OH)_2\ (aq) + H_2\ (g)$$

In a double-displacement reactions two compounds swap components $(AB + CD \rightarrow AD + CB)$.

$$Na_2S\ (aq) + 2HCl\ (aq) \rightarrow 2NaCl\ (aq) + H_2S\ (g)$$
$$BaCl_2\ (aq) + H_2SO_4\ (aq) \rightarrow BaSO_4\ (s) + 2HCl\ (aq)$$
$$KOH\ (aq) + HNO_3\ (aq) \rightarrow H_2O\ (l) + KNO_3\ (aq)$$

In a precipitation reaction the reactants exchange ions to form an insoluble salt.

$$BaCl_2\ (aq) + Na_2SO_4\ (aq) \rightarrow BaSO_4\ (s) + 2NaCl\ (aq)$$
$$Ba^{2+}\ (aq),\ Cl^-\ (aq),\ Na^+\ (aq),\ \text{and}\ SO_4^{2-}\ (aq)$$

Another type of double-displacement reaction occurs when an insoluble gas is formed.

$$ZnS\ (s) + 2HCl\ (aq) \rightarrow ZnCl_2\ (aq) + H_2S\ (g)$$
$$H_2CO_3\ (aq) \rightarrow H_2O\ (l) + CO_2\ (g)$$
$$CaCO_3\ (s) + 2HCl\ (aq) \rightarrow CaCl_2\ (aq) + H_2CO_3\ (aq)$$
$$CaCO_3\ (s) + 2HCl\ (aq) \rightarrow CaCl_2\ (aq) + H_2O\ (l) + CO_2\ (g)$$

Acid-base neutralisation reactions are a kind of double-displacement reaction of an acid and a base.

$$HCl\ (aq) + NaOH\ (aq) \rightarrow NaCl\ (aq) + H_2O\ (l)$$

Spot the Difference

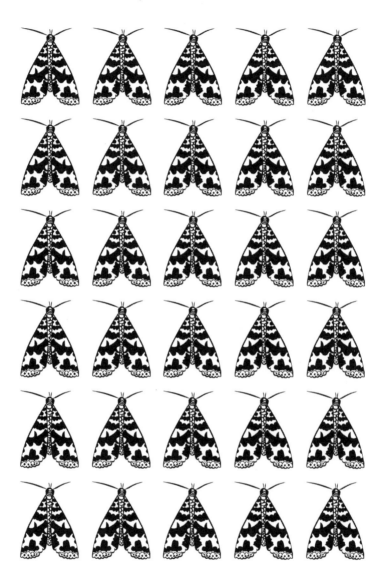

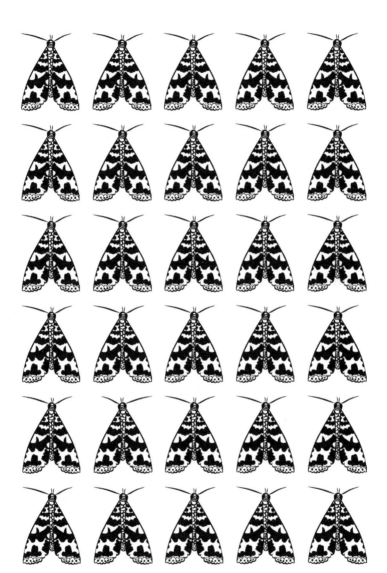

The Morphology of Roots and Tubers of the Andes

There are at least 25 species of tuber and root crops in South America, across 16 botanical genera and 15 families, which include a variety of monocotyledons and dicotyledons. A morphological approach to the Andean roots and tubers is not necessarily an easy task since in many respects the various species are quite dissimilar: they exhibit, for instance, varying botanical families, life-forms, propagation methods and chemical compositions. However, they do mostly have the common characteristic of being perennial underground plants, with the exception of biennial maca (see below).

The roots and tubers are mostly found across three altitudinally defined phytogeographic zones: the cool-temperate highlands are found at an altitude of about 2,500 to 4,000 metres; at about 1,000 to 2,500 metres altitude we find the subtropical zone, in valleys between the Andean mountains; and from 4,000 metres up to the highest points at which cultivation is feasible (about 4,500 metres) we find the intensely cold sub-arctic puna.

These roots and tubers are mainly used in remote rural communities, where a principal use is for starch extraction – or for their leaves only (which are used as wrappers while the root or tuber is left to rot in the ground). Fewer than a million Andean people actually eat the roots and tubers, and the numbers are declining. Most ahipa and mauka farmers have, for instance, given up growing the crops entirely. Before considering the morphological distinctions and resemblances between the various species, here is a brief introduction to some of the roots and tubers:

Oca (*Oxalis tuberosa*) is a widely cultivated tuber. It can be white or greyish, contains amino acids, fibre and antioxidants and can be boiled over a long period to create a stew or soup. It is fairly flavourless and prone to being attacked by the oca weevil.

Ulluco (*Ullucus tuberosus*) is another tuber of the Andean region. It comes in various colours and shapes. It contains protein, calcium and other chemical components. It can be boiled over a period of several hours or days to create a fairly flavourless stew or soup. Another tuber, mashua (*Tropaeolum tuberosum*), can be white or other colours. It contains levels of isothiocyanates (glucosinolates), and can be boiled over a period of hours or days to create a fairly flavourless stew. The Incas mainly recommended it for the purpose of dampening down sexual desires.

Yacón (*Smallanthus sonchifolius*) is another tuber of the Andean region. It has a white or off-white colour, contains oligofructose, and can be eaten raw, although some locals prefer to boil it for several days until it has become a flavourless soup or stew. Ahipa is another root that can be eaten raw in particular situations. It is a legume root produced by the yam bean (*Pachyrhizus*) and contains alkaloids and rotenone in its seeds, stems and leaves, which makes the seeds, in particular, inedible. As well as eating the non-toxic parts of the plant raw, Andean locals boil it for a few hours to produce a flavourless stew.

Maca is the only cruciferae that has been domesticated in the Andean region. It can be a variety of colours, including white and off-white. It mainly survives in inhospitable environments and contains glucosinolates. It can be boiled for days or hours to produce a variety of soups and stews of little flavour or interest. Arracacha (*Arracacia xanthorrhiza*) is another root of the Andean region. It is susceptible to viruses, so has to be eaten reasonably soon after it has been harvested. It has a dense flesh that resembles the flesh of some of the other tubers and roots of the Andean region. It can be boiled over long periods or added to stews and soups. Achira (*Canna edulis*), which can also be called edible canna or Queensland arrowroot, is a rhizome with large starch granules, of various colours. Ancient Peruvians used it as a staple, boiling it for days in order to produce a soup or stew. Further morphological complexities are still being analyzed.

The Life and Works of Porphyry the Neoplatonist

Porphyry was born in Phoenicia in Tyre sometime in the early third century AD. He can be referred to as 'Malcus', or the more common appellation 'Porphyry'. In his twenties he studied under the Middle Platonist Longinus. However, he then went on to study with Plotinus in Rome. Either or both of Plotinus and Porphyry have been credited as the originator of the school of Neoplatonism. Porphyry edited *The Enneads*, the collected works of Plotinus, which consists of six books each containing nine treatises. He also wrote over 60 works, many of which are now lost or forgotten. Three of the surviving manuscripts and texts are *Starting-points Leading to the Intelligibles* (also known as the *Sententiae* or *Sententiae ad Intelligibilia Ducentes*), the *Isagoge* (Introduction), and *To Gaurus*.

Porphyry's philosophical views were also influenced by Longinus, Numenius and other Middle Platonists, as is shown by *Sententiae ad Intelligibilia Ducentes*. Both Plotinus and Porphyry wrote about the three 'hypostases' (different ontological levels). In this view of ontological questions there is a distinction between the sensible realm, the intellect and the intelligible, and humanity is identified with the intellect as well as with the intelligible.

For Porphyry the hierarchy of hypostases contains the One, Intellect and Soul, in a metaphysical framework that is substantially similar to the metaphysical framework that will be familiar to readers from the works of Plotinus. Some academics have identified Porphyry's concept of the One as a kind of ineffable first principle that distinguishes it from the definition of the One in the works of Plotinus. But if we take this view the distinction between the first and the second of the three hypostases becomes harder to define. Suggesting that the ineffable One be treated this way consequently seems somewhat un-Porphyrian.

A few fragments of *Ad Gedalium*, a commentary by Porphyry on the works of Aristotle, survive, alongside the *Isagoge*, which also refers to Aristotle's logic, metaphysics and epistemology. The *Isagoge* is thus a key work in the development of Neoplatonism, especially with respect to the interaction between epistemology and the three hypostases.

Porphyry's writing on Aristotle is distinguished from Plotinus in its suggestion that particulars should be treated as prior to universals. Aristotelian categories such as substance, quality and quantity would thus be treated not in primary ontological terms but as part of the sensible realm. Academics who have written commentaries on Neoplatonist thought have varying views on how this could be taken to affect the basic ontology, but tend to agree that the realm of Platonic Forms can be related to the intelligible universals if not always directly to the sensible realm.

As well as his interesting and nuanced relationship with the ontology and epistemology of Aristotle and Plotinus, Porphyry wrote a commentary on the Chaldean Oracles, a second-century religious text revered by certain Neoplatonists, including Iamblichus. Following in his wake, post-Iamblichean Neoplatonism regarded religion, religious rites and theurgy as potential routes to salvation. Iamblichus (who can also be referred to as Iamblichus of Apamea or Iamblichus Chalcidensis) was a contemporary Neoplatonist. His work *Protrepticus* is well known for having preserved some of the works of Anonymous Iamblichi, a name given to the unknown sophist whose works are quoted by Iamblichus in *Protrepticus*. The name 'Anonymous' is of course deliberately chosen to draw attention to his anonymity.

Porphyry had some significant doctrinal differences with Iamblichus; in particular he criticised the latter's views on theurgy. Iamblichus responded to these criticisms in his work *De Mysteriis Aegyptiorum*. Iamblichus also placed the One at the head of an ordering of hypostases, although he then added an additional superexistent 'One' between this One and the many, creating a preliminary dyad rather than a triad of hypostases.

Waste Disposal: a Global Guide

- The guide to sorting your garbage for recycling in Niihama City in Japan is 21 pages long.

- In New Zealand the Waste Management Hierarchy policy was incorporated into national law in the Local Government Amendment Act No.4, 1996.

- Estonia met its 2013 target for bio-degradable municipal waste being sent to landfill ahead of schedule in 2009.

- In South Africa the volume of waste generated in 1997 was about 500 million tons.

- Denmark incinerates approximately 80 per cent of its household waste.

- Waste disposal in Portugal is one of the administrative tasks that has been devolved to the municipal authorities.

- In 2013 Belgium was announced as the best-performing country in waste management in the EU.

- Waste disposal in Liechtenstein is regulated by the Act on Environmental Protection (29 May 2008) – comparable to the Swiss Federal Act on Protection, which sets out basic standards for the handling of waste and contaminated sites.

- In Minnesota the statute MS s 115A.914 sets out the technical standards that a responsible collector of used tyres must adhere to.

- In Vietnam the Prime Minister's Decision 1929/QD-TTg on the 'Orientation for Development of Water Supply in Vietnam's Urban Centres and Industrial Parks Leading to 2025, and Vision for 2050' set out a target of reducing the rate of water loss in named cities to less than 15 per cent by 2025.

- In Latvia there are more than 3,000 commercial or educational institutions that provide special containers for collecting worn-out batteries.

- The recycling project in Barbados has been managed by the Government of Barbados's Solid Waste Project Unit in co-operation with the Sustainable Barbados Recycling Centre (SBRC).

- In Saudi Arabia the per capita generation of waste in 2015 was approximately 1.5 to 1.8 kilograms per person per day.

The Evolution of the Airbag:
Key Dates and Events

- 1952: John W. Hetrick proposes the idea of the airbag after having been in a car accident.

- 1953: Hetrick receives a patent for 'a safety cushion assembly for automotive vehicles'.

- 1953: German inventor Walter Linderer receives a similar patent for an inflatable device to cushion drivers in accidents.

- Late 1950s: Ford and General Motors start experimental work on airbags.

- 1963: Japanese inventor, Yasuzaburou Kobori, designs a reliable system for triggering a quick-release burst of compressed air.

- 1966: Ford and Eaton, Yale & Towne both attempt to use a military detonating valve to trigger an airbag.

- 1967: Crash sensors using a magnet and ball system are designed.

- 1967: Airbags using sodium azide and other non-oxygen gases are introduced.

- Late 1960s: Mechanic Allen K. Breed invents a reliable, $5 crash sensor.

- 1969: U.S. federal laws require 'automatic occupant protection systems' for all new cars sold.

- Early 1970s: Airbags are offered as an experimental extra in some Ford, General Motors and Chrysler cars, as well as in some European models.

- 1970s: Ford plans to use airbags in an entire new production line, but then abandons the plan.

- 1973: The Oldsmobile Toronado is the first car to offer a passenger airbag.

- 1973: General Motors installs an alternative airbag in the Chevrolet Impala but the line fails and they abandon their airbag plans.

- 1974: Buick, Cadillac and Oldsmobile offer dual airbags on various lines of their cars.

- 1980: Mercedes-Benz in Germany offers the airbag as an option for their model W126.

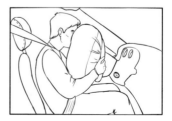

Comparative Rates of Reproduction
in Insect Pests

Farmers and ecologists are among those who can benefit from a full understanding of the comparative rates of reproduction in insect pests. There are, of course, many factors that can affect such rates of reproduction. Density-independent factors include factors such as extremes of weather, humidity and dissolved oxygen for water-borne pests. Density-dependent factors include factors such as disease, intra-population competition and inter-population competition, as well as migration. When studying population dynamics we also need to take into account factors such as birth, mortality, reproductive success and individual growth. We also have to take into account whether a species has a life cycle that is semelparous or iteroparous. An iteroparous species is one that can have multiple reproductive events within its life cycle, while a semelparous species is one that does not. However, the two categories are not entirely clear-cut, as some semelparous species can theoretically be classified as partially iteroparous and vice versa depending on definition and context.

In order to compare the rates of reproduction in various species, we use life tables, which keep track of such factors as births, deaths and reproductive output. We can construct life tables in different forms: as cohort life tables, detailing the data on a group of same-aged individuals through their lives from birth to death; as a static life table based on data collected from an entire population at one time; or as a variant form of life table constructed from mortality data in a particular period.

To construct a cohort life table for an iteroparous species of insect pest we first estimate the population size from methods such as the capture-capture method in which two samples of the population are caught at different times and compared to one another after the operatives have marked the first set of captured insects and released them back into the population. We then construct a table starting with columns for the age classification of individuals, the number alive at a certain age (l_x) – we can then use the remaining columns for a variety of calculations concerning the proportions of individuals surviving and not surviving at various stages of the life cycle of the species.

For instance, the subsequent columns for a life table for a white-fly population would be: portion of original sample dying during each stage (d_x); mortality rate (q_x); eggs produced at each stage (F_x); eggs produced per surviving individual at each stage (m_x); and eggs produced per original individual in each stage $(l_x m_x)$.

Having constructed this table we can move on to make a variety of calculations about the expected mortality of original individuals, surviving individuals and the reproductive rate of individual members of the population and the population as a whole. For instance, to calculate life expectancy we use this method. For the average proportion D_x, of individuals alive at each stage x we add l_x to l_{x+1} and then divide the sum of the two figures by 2. So, obviously, the total number T_x of future stages that we would expect to be lived by individuals at the age of x is $l_x + l_{x+1} + l_{x+2} \ldots$ And from this we can calculate the life expectancy e_x by dividing the latter sum by l_x.

Next, assuming we know the number of eggs produced at each stage (F_x), and the number of surviving individuals (a_x), we can calculate the eggs produced per remaining individual of the original population (m_x) by dividing the former by the latter. Now we get to the really crucial part of the calculations, the basic reproductive rate or replacement rate of a population (R_o). It should be clear that each measurement of $l_x m_x$ is simply a calculation of first-generation parents at age x divided by first-generation eggs multiplied by the second-generation eggs produced by parents of age x then divided by the first-generation parents at age x. So we simply take the sum of the $l_x m_x$ elements to find R_o.

A History of Early Carpet Manufacture in the United States of America

- The first woven carpet mill was opened in Philadelphia in 1791.

- More carpet mills were opened during the early 1800s.

- In 1839 Erastus Bigelow invented a power loom for carpet weaving. It is known as 'Bigelow's loom'.

- Alexander Smith opened a carpet manufacturing plant in 1845 in New York State.

- Jacquard mechanisms were first used in power looms in 1849.

- The modified Brussels loom was subsequently used in the manufacture of Wilton carpets.

- The Bigelow Carpet Company was formed by a merger between Hartford Carpet Company and Clinton Company in 1864.

- In 1876 Halcyon Skinner, who had developed a method of manufacturing Royal Axminster, combined his company with that of Alexander Smith's to form Alexander Smith & Sons.

- Erastus Bigelow (see above) was also responsible for the first broadloom carpet in 1877, as well as many other innovations he introduced into the field of carpet manufacture.

- In 1878 the Shuttleworth Brothers Company opened in New York State.

- In the late nineteenth century tufted carpet was developed as a cottage industry in the region of Dalton, Georgia. By the end of the century there were over 10,000 tufters working in the region.

- In 1900, inspired partly by the tufted carpets of the Dalton region, Catherine Evans Whitener sold her first handcrafted bedspread for $2.50. She would go on to sell many more.

- In 1905 the Shuttleworth Brothers Company premiered a new carpet, the Karnak Wilton.

- In 1920 Mohawk Carpet Mills was formed following a merger between Shuttleworth Brothers Company and McCleary, Wallin and Crouse, who were also a carpet manufacturer in the same region.

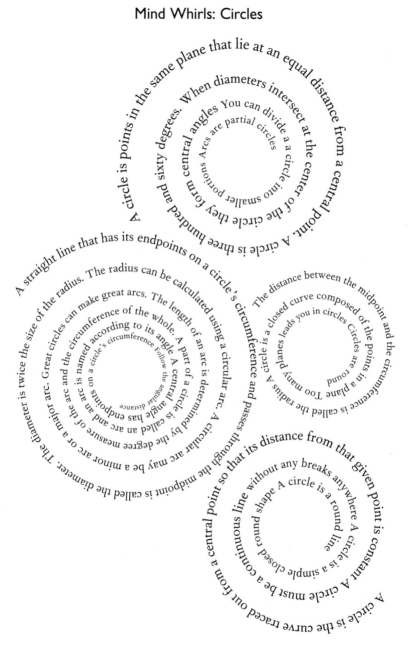

A circle is points in the same plane that lie at an equal distance from a central point. A circle is three hundred and sixty degrees. When diameters intersect at the center of the circle they form central angles You can divide a circle into smaller portions Arcs are partial circles

A straight line that has its endpoints on a circle's circumference and passes through the midpoint is called the diameter. The diameter is twice the size of the radius. The radius can be calculated using a circular arc. A circular arc may be a minor arc or a major arc. Great circles can make great arcs. The length of an arc is determined by the degree measure of the arc and an arc is named according to its angle A central angle has endpoints on a circle's circumference follow the angular distance the circumference of the whole. A part of a circle is called an arc and the

The distance between the midpoint and the circumference is called the radius Circles are round Too many planes leads you in circles A circle is a closed curve composed of the points in a plane

A circle is the curve traced out from a central point so that its distance from that given point is constant A circle must be a continuous line without any breaks anywhere A circle is a round line A circle is a simple closed round shape A circle is a round

Iambic Pentameter and
Some Other Metres

Prosody is the study of the patterns of rhyme and sound in poetry. The metre of a line of poetry is the fundamental rhythmic structure of a verse or lines in verse. Iambic pentameter, the most frequently used metre in English poetry, is a line that uses five feet (a foot being a smaller group of syllables). An iamb is a particular type of foot in which an unstressed syllable is followed by a stressed syllable so, obviously, a line made up of five iambs is described as iambic pentameter.

Similar schemes have been used in other European languages, with the modification that the only fixed stressed syllable is the one that comes at the end of the pattern. This kind of metre is called a qualitative metre as opposed to quantitative metre, in which the weight of the syllable matters more than the number of syllables. In Latin and Greek poetry of the classical period dactylic hexameter was made up of six feet, each of which was either a spondee or a dactyl (the difference being based on whether the syllables in the foot were long or short, rather than whether they were stressed or unstressed). Sanskrit and classical Arabic used similar metres.

Languages without strong stresses, including Chinese and French, tend to use metres that are more closely based on the number of syllables. In France the alexandrine is commonly used – this involves two hemstitchs (a hemstitch is half a line) of six syllables each, with a caesura, or a word-break, in the middle. The alexandrine isn't quite as ubiquitous in French verse as the iambic pentameter in English verse: for instance, early French poets often used the *décasyllabe* and *octosyllabe* while more modern poets started to experiment with the structure of the hemstitches. It is also important to bear in mind that some types of metre are less easy to identify. Vedic metre and Sanskrit metre use feet, but it is not always possible to distinguish a foot from a line: in Sanskrit syllabic verse (*akṣasravṛtta*) the metres are defined by the number of syllables in a verse, while in syllabo-quantitative verse (*vaṇavṛtta*) metres depend on syllable count in a different way. In Greek and Latin poetry, as well as dactylic hexameter, an important metre was the dactylic pentameter, which could be in the form an elegiac distich or elegiac couplet. Meanwhile, in Aeolic verse the hendeca-syllabic line (with 11 syllables) was often deployed to great effect.

In Spanish poetry the use of poetic licences, in which the num-ber of syllables in the line varies, must be taken into account, in particular syneresis, dieresis, synalepha and hiatus. The most com-mon actual metres used in Spanish are septenary (a 7-syllable line), octosyllable (an 8-syllable line), hendecasyllable (an 11-syllable line) and alexandrine. Note that while in French or English poetry the alexandrine is a 12-syllable line separated into two hemstitches, in Spanish poetry it is a 14-syllable line separated into two hem-stitches.

In Italian poetry the definitions change once again as the rhythm of the language favours the use of a paroxytone, in which the penultimate syllable is stressed. As a result a septenary (which would in Spanish, of course, contain seven syllables) will have a stress on the sixth syllable but could contain six, seven or eight syllables. (Italian poetry mostly avoids the use of a novenary, with nine syllables.)

When it comes to Portuguese poetry there are further compli-cations. A *redondilha menor* is made up of five syllables, while a *redondilha maior* is made up of seven syllables, as in a traditional septenary. The *decassílabo* is the equivalent of a decasyllable and uses 10 syllables. The *dodecassílabo* (dodecasyllable) is made up of 12 syllables and can also take the form of an alexandrine in which the two hemstitches have 6 syllables each. Portuguese poetry addi-tionally uses *bárbaro* (lines made up of 13 or more syllables) and *lucasiano*, which is similar to the alexandrine but is composed of 16 syllables split into two hemstitches of 8 syllables each.

Lentils: the Healthy Option

Lentils are a food source that combines a high protein content with a wide variety of health benefits. They are a good source of crucial amino acids, including isoleucine and lysine. In addition, sprouted lentils contain the amino acids methionine and cysteine. They also contain a wide variety of minerals and vitamins, as well as fibre. Their proportion of carbohydrates is up to 25 grams per 100 grams. They also contain vitamin B1, folate, molybdenum, iron, tryptophan, manganese, phosphorous, copper and potassium, as well as a variety of phytochemicals and phenols. Let's take a specific look at some of their health benefits.

One aspect of your lifestyle that lentils can help with is in maintaining a healthy heart. Of course, lentils on their own aren't sufficient to foster good health in this respect. Other important tips are to give up smoking, if you are a smoker, be more active, stay at or attain a healthy weight, cut down on saturated fat, eat a balanced diet with lots of fruit and vegetables, cut down on salt to avoid high blood pressure, and to substitute fish for meat (if you are a meat-eater).

The main dangers you face if you don't maintain a healthy heart are coronary artery disease, heart failure and heart attack. These have slightly different symptoms. The symptoms of coronary heart disease include angina, shortness of breath, palpitations, tachycardia, dizziness, nausea and sweating. The symptoms of a heart attack include discomfort or pain in the chest, below the breastbone or in the arm (this pain may also spread to the back, jaw, throat or hand), indigestion or heartburn, sweating, nausea, dizziness, weakness and anxiety, and tachycardia or irregular heartbeats. If you believe you are having a heart attack it is important to seek medical advice as fast as possible. Symptoms of arrhythmia (an abnormal heart rhythm) may also include palpitations, pounding in the chest, dizziness, fainting, shortness of breath, discomfort in the chest and fatigue.

Of course, fatigue is not necessarily a symptom of an unhealthy heart, so it is important to consider what other causes it may have and also the consequences of fatigue. Fatigue can lead to chronic sleepiness, headaches, sore muscles, dizziness, delayed responses, poor decisionmaking, poor hand-to-eye coordination, appetite loss, irritability, blurry vision, memory loss, hallucination, poor concentration, low motivation, poor concentration, listlessness, world-weariness, tiredness, boredom, lassitude, difficulty keeping your eyes open, confusion, uncertainty, clumsiness, muscle weakness, poor concentration, and many other problems.

So why would you be suffering from fatigue? Well, some of the reasons might be: coeliac disease, which is a food intolerance, where your body has a bad reaction to gluten, which is found in pies, cakes, wheat, beer, bread, breadsticks, scones, many biscuits, ale, pastry, bread rolls and other types of food; anaemia, which is iron deficiency, a problem that affects around 5 per cent of men and a proportion of women post-menopause and which leads to tiredness, lassitude and a heavy feeling; chronic fatigue syndrome (myalgic encephalomyelitis, or ME), a debilitating illness which can last for months or years and causes aching limbs, inflamed glands, tiredness, muscle pain, migraine, sore throat and a variety of other symptoms; sleep apnoea, in which your throat closes slightly during sleep, interrupting your breathing and waking you up; an underactive thyroid gland, meaning that you have a deficiency of thyroid hormone (thyroxine), which is likely to lead to tiredness, weight gain, aching muscles and lassitude; diabetes, a long-term illness that can be diagnosed with a blood test, and which is caused by an excess of blood sugar, so tends to require changes in diet and lifestyle; and glandular fever, which is a viral infection that causes fever, swollen glands and a sore throat in the first instance, but which can leave you feeling tired and weary and weak for months afterwards.

How Rocks Become Pebbles

- Pebbles are a particular type of geological formation and appearance that is formed over a period of time.

- In the sea, various types of rock are gradually eroded until they become elliptical, rounded or flatter than normal rocks.

- The axis around which a pebble can most easily rotate will define how the process of erosion shapes it over time. For instance, rocks that start as ellipses will become more elliptical over time as the ocean water moves them around and rotates individual pebbles against other pebbles.

- The typical size range of a pebble is from about 2.5 millimetres to 45 millimetres, but some pebbles are as large as 10 to 15 centimetres.

- Pebbles come in different colours, ranging from translucent white to black, and shades of yellow, brown, red and green.

- Sea pebbles of any size often tend to have an ellipsoidal shape, but can also look like eggs.

- Non-ellipsoidal pebbles can often be flat or spherical.

- A spherical pebble will roll through the water more easily than an ellipsoidal or flat pebble.

- Pebbles are rarely square because their corners get eroded by water.

- Sea pebbles are found on beaches of most oceans and seas, and also inland where seas have receded from an area of land.

- The coasts of the Pacific Ocean have some especially plentiful pebble beaches, but there are also pebble beaches in northern Europe (especially in the Norwegian Sea) and around Australia, Indonesia and Japan as well as other areas of the world.

- Pebbles also form inland in rivers, lakes and ponds, where they are technically known as inland pebbles or river pebbles.

- The smoothness and colour of river pebbles depends on a variety of factors, including the type of rock, the soil of the river bed and the speed of the current.

- River currents aren't as strong as ocean waves, so river pebbles are usually not as smooth as beach pebbles (although some river pebbles will be carried by currents into the ocean, where they will become sea pebbles).

Sleeping in History

- In *Poimandres: The Vision* the ancient Hermetic writer Hermes Trismegistus wrote that the 'sleep of the body is the sober watchfulness of the Mind and the shutting of my eyes reveals the true Light'.

- Napoleon Bonaparte recommended six hours' sleep per day for a man, seven for a woman and eight for a fool. He ended being deposed and exiled.

- Leonardo da Vinci was a polyphasic sleeper, meaning that he slept only in short regular bursts.

- The Hippocratic text *On Regimine* (fifth century BC) suggests that a daily nap in the afternoon is good for your health.

- The Emperor Charlemagne liked to take a nap for several hours in the afternoon.

- The National Association of Friends of the Siesta holds championships in Spain to celebrate their somnambulist heritage.

- The ancient physician Galen believed you could diagnose illnesses from dreams, which he referred to as the vision-in-sleep (enhypnion). For instance, he argued that dreaming of a confla-gration could indicate a problem with your yellow bile.

- Rufus of Ephesus also wrote about the importance of dreams in medical diagnosis, as did the ancient Greek writer Herophilos, allegedly.

- Hippocratic physicians also focused on the question of dreams and the health or ill health of the patient. However, they were more interested in the frequency of the occurrence of dreams rather than their contents.

- In the 1990s the psychiatrist Thomas Wehr conducted a study in which he placed subjects in total darkness for 14 hours a day for a month.

- Until the seventeenth to eighteen centuries, when electric lighting and an increase in consumption of caffeine changed our lifestyles, many people would have two sessions of sleep a day rather than one overnight session. This is known as dual sleeping.

- In the dream cult of Asclepius, pilgrims in need of healing or spiritual guidance spent a night sleeping in the temple of Asclepius and then told the priest what they had dreamed about.

The Distances between Galaxies

When measuring the distances between galaxies, astronomers use a variety of methods. Firstly, bear in mind that while we often talk about light-years, the more technical term preferred in astronomy is the parsec, which is 3.26 light-years or, to be precise, the distance at which one astronomical unit subtends an angle of one second of arc. For larger distances we can use the kiloparsec (kpc) or megaparsec (mpc). From one side to the other of the Milky Way is about 100,000 light-years or 30 kiloparsecs – the solar system is about 8 kiloparsecs from the centre of the galaxy.

When calculating greater distances, such as those between separate galaxies, astronomers use a variety of methods. For instance: parallaxes, proper motions, moving clusters, interstellar lines using absorption lines in the spectrum, the inverse-square law (which states that the flux from a luminous object decreases as the square of its distance), the period-luminosity relation (which depends on the fact that for stars that are regular pulsators, the period of one oscillation is related to their luminosity), or methods such as using radio telescopes to observe the wavelength of neutral hydrogen gas or carbon monoxide.

Using a variety of these methods astronomers have concluded that the Canis Major Dwarf galaxy, whose status as a galaxy is of course disputed, is about 0.008 megaparsecs from the Earth. Beyond that we reach the Sagittarius Dwarf Spheroidal galaxy at about 0.024 megaparsecs. Ursa Major II Dwarf galaxy is 25 per cent further away at 0.03 megaparsecs, while the Large Magellanic Cloud is 0.05 megaparsecs away. Next, we reach Boötes I galaxy at 0.06 megaparsecs away, although obviously when we say next, we mean next in the list of distant galaxies, as these galaxies are not all in the same direction. Indeed, most of them lie in completely different directions so that the difficulty of arranging to visit more than one of them would be extremely great.

The Small Magellanic Cloud is 0.063 megaparsecs away, as is the Ursa Minor Dwarf galaxy. (Incidentally, dwarf galaxies are still very large, just not as large as galaxies that aren't so-called.) Then there is a gap to another dwarf, the Draco Dwarf galaxy at 0.079 megaparsecs, then NGC 2419 at 0.084 megaparsecs. Sextans Dwarf Spheroidal galaxy is 0.086 megaparsecs away. Sculptor Dwarf galaxy is 0.088 megaparsecs, then the next galaxy is 0.1 megaparsecs away – this is Ursa Major Dwarf galaxy. At the same distance from the Earth, but in a different direction, we find the Carina Dwarf galaxy, then the Fornax Dwarf galaxy is 0.14 megaparsecs away.

Between that distance and half a megaparsec away we find the following galaxies: Leo II Dwarf (0.21 megaparsecs), Leo I Dwarf (0.25 megaparsecs), Leo T Dwarf (0.42 megaparsecs), Phoenix Dwarf galaxy (0.44 megaparsecs) and Barnard's galaxy (0.5 megaparsecs). Bear in mind that half a megaparsec is over one and a half million light-years, meaning that when we see light from Barnard's galaxy it has been travelling for over one and a half million years to reach the Earth. If we were to actually travel there it would, of course, take much longer, since we are unable to travel at or even near to the speed of light.

Beyond half a megaparsec there is an increase in the number of galaxies that aren't named other than with a sequence of letters and numbers because, frankly, astronomers don't have much imagination when it comes to nomenclature. So we get MGC 1 (which can be described either as a globular cluster or a galaxy) at 0.61 megaparsecs away, NGC 185 at 0.62 megaparsecs away, Andromeda II (which has a name, but not a new one, because, as we will see below, there are other galaxies called Andromeda) at 0.65 megaparsecs away, IC 10 at 0.67 megaparsecs away, NGC 147 at 0.68 megaparsces away, IC 1613 at 0.72 megaparsecs away, Andromeda I, Andromeda III and Cetus Dwarf galaxies.

The Caesar Cipher
Explained and Explicated

The Caesar Cipher is an early example of a code or cipher, which was apparently used by Julius Caesar to encrypt his secret messages. It is based on a very simple principle, which is to substitute each letter of the plaintext message with a letter a given number of letters ahead in the alphabet. For this reason it is also an example of a substitution cipher. For instance, if you are encrypting the message 'the quick brown fox jumps over the lazy dog' and using a rot1 shift (meaning that you rotate by 1 place through the alphabet) the ciphertext will be 'uif rvjdl cspxo gpy kvnqt pwfs uif mbaz eph' or, if you prefer to arrange the message in groups of three letters and omit the capital letters to make the message marginally harder to decrypt, 'uif rvjd lcsp xog pyk vnq tpw fsu ifm baz eph'. If you were to use a rot2 shift instead of a rot1 shift then the same message would be encrypted as 'vjg swkem dtqyp hqz lworu qxgt vjg ncba fqi'. Or if you use a rot3 shift it would be encrypted as 'wkh txlfn eurzq ira mxpsv ryhu wkh odcb grj'.

Incidentally, the sentence 'the quick brown fox jumps over the lazy dog' is an example of a pangram, a sentence or piece of text that uses every letter of the alphabet, which is why it is a good example to use when demonstrating the use of the Caesar Cipher. Some other examples of short pangrams are 'jived fox nymph grabs quick waltz', 'glib jocks quiz nymph to vex dwarf', 'sphinx of black quartz, judge my vow', 'the five boxing wizards jump quickly', 'pack my box with five dozen liquor jugs' and 'how vexingly quick daft zebras jump'!

A variation on the pangram is the self-enumerating pangram, which counts its own letters. For instance, the sentence 'this pangram contains four As, one B, two Cs, one D, thirty Es, six Fs, five Gs, seven Hs, eleven Is, one J, one K, two Ls, two Ms, eighteen

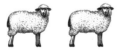

Ns, fifteen Os, two Ps, one Q, five Rs, twenty-seven Ss, eighteen Ts, two Us, seven Vs, eight Ws, two Xs, three Ys & one Z' contains every letter of the alphabet and is also an accurate inventory of the number of letters in the sentence itself. (Mathematically speaking, self-enumerating pangrams can be reduced to the Boolean satisfiability problem: this has been demonstrated by using hardware description language and the Tseytin transformation.) Self-enumerating pangrams are, in turn, an example of autograms, sentences that describe their own contents. (Whereas reflexicons are pairs of sentences that accurately describe each other's contents.) If we take the sentence above and put it through a rot4 Caesar shift we get this sentence: 'Xlmw terkveq gsrxemrw jsyv Ew, sri F, xas Gw, sri H, xlmvxc Iw, wmb Jw, jmzi Kw, wizir Lw, ipizir Mw, sri N, sri O, xas Pw, xas Qw, imklxiir Rw, jmjxiir Sw, xas Tw, sri U, jmzi Vw, xairxc-wizir Ww, imklxiir Xw, xas Yw, wizir Zw, imklx Aw, xas Bw, xlvii Cw & sri D'. This highlights a significant and serious problem with Caesar shift encryption of autograms: the original sentence uses the letters of the alphabet in an easily observed sequence, which makes it too easy to guess what rotation has been used in the substitution cipher. However, this problem is not insurmountable. One solution would be to encrypt the sentence differently, by moving the inventory of letters back around to the correct order: 'Xlmw terkveq gsrxemrw imklx Aw, xas Bw, xlvii Cw, sri D, jsyv Ew, sri F, xas Gw, sri H, xlmvxc Iw, wmb Jw, jmzi Kw, wizir Lw, ipizir Mw, sri N, sri O, xas Pw, xas Qw, imklxiir Rw, jmjxiir Sw, xas Tw, sri U, jmzi Vw, xairxc-wizir Ww, imklxiir Xw, xas Yw & wizir Zw'. When we decrypt this the message is slightly garbled: 'This pangram contains eight Ws, two Xs, three Ys, one Z, four As, one B, two Cs, one D, thirty Es, six Fs, five Gs, seven Hs, eleven Is, one J, one K, two Ls, two Ms, eighteen Ns, fifteen Os, two Ps, one Q, five Rs, twenty-seven Ss, eighteen Ts, two Us & seven Vs'. But this is still an autogram, and it would be easy for the receiver of the message to rearrange the inventory of letters back into the correct order.

Brief Historical Anecdotes Concerning
the History of the Harlequinade

- On New Year's night in 1091 a priest called Gauchelin reported having been startled by a wild hunt parade, which may or may not have been an early incarnation of the Harlequinade.

- During the Middle Ages, in theatrical appearances, 'Herlekin' was generally accompanied by his troupe, the Mesnie Herlekin.

- The Harlequinade is possibly mentioned in *Jeu de la Feuillée* by Adam de la Halle when the character Morgue refers to his master Hellequin.

- The character Arlecchino, who appears in Italian masques, and who was associated with the Bergamesque dance, is another possible forerunner of Harlequin.

- The outrageous rogueries of the Harlequins are also mentioned in the *Recueil Fossard*, a set of pictorial documents related to festivities in the court of Louis XIV.

- Harlequin the clown is mentioned in '*Histoire plaisante des faicts et gestes de Harlequin commedien Italien contenant ses songes et visions, etc.*', two French poems published in 1585.

- The early clown Tristan Martinelli was also known as Arlechinus or Dominus Arlechinorum.

- The sayings of another Harlequin, Giuseppe-Domenico Biancolelli, also known as Dominique, were collected by C. Cotolendi in a book called *Arlequiniana*.

- In the seventeenth-century play *Arlequin lingère du Palais,* Harlequin appears in a costume that is partially based on that of a laundress and partially based on that of a lemonade seller.

- The Bohemian actor Jean-Gaspard Deburau only played Harlequin after Felix the Harlequin of the Funambules allowed him to take over the role, previously played by Felix himself.

- In 1847 Paul Legrand took the role of Pierrot at the Funambules and, together with his well-known colleague Champfleury, introduced an increasing level of macabre menace into the role of Harlequin.

Mind Whirls: Washing Cycles

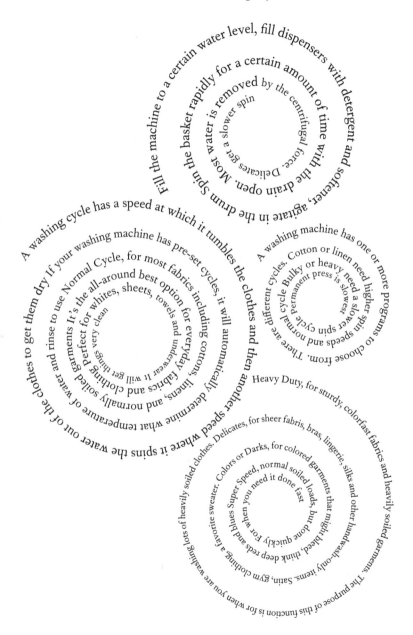

The Paradox of the Grain of Millet

A less well-known paradox from the philosopher Zeno is the paradox of the grain of millet. The basic statement of this paradox is that when you drop a single grain of millet to the ground it makes no sound, whereas if you drop a thousand grains of millet to the ground they do make a noise. This implies that if you add together a thousand nothings then you have something, which appears to be an absurdity. Aristotle attempted to refute this by pointing out that 'there is no reason why any such part should not in any length of time fail to move the air that the whole bushel moves in falling . . . in fact it does not of itself move even such a quantity of the air as it would move if this part were by itself: for no part even exists otherwise than potentially'. Others have pointed out that this is essentially a Parmenidean argument because Aristotle is suggesting rather than seeing the situation as many nothings adding up to a something, we should see it as many inaudible things adding up to an audible thing, which is incrementally different. One is reminded of *The Analyst* by Bishop Berkeley in which he attempts to refute the art of calculus using not dissimilar arguments, which one might consider Zenoesque. Berkeley considers the increments that we discard at the exact moment of calculation during a differentiation calculation, arguing that this is a 'fallacious way of proceeding to a certain Point on the Supposition of an Increment, and then at once shifting your Supposition to that of no Increment . . . Since if this second Supposition had been made before the common Division by [the increment], all had vanished at once, and you must have got nothing by your Supposition. Whereas by this Artifice of first dividing, and then changing your Supposition, you retain 1 and nxn-1. But, notwithstanding all this address to cover it, the fallacy is still the same'. Berkeley goes on to reject Newton's concept of fluxions, which are of course a kind of increment, thus: 'And what are these Fluxions? The Velocities of evanescent Increments? And what are these same evanescent Increments? They are neither finite Quantities nor Quantities infinitely small, nor yet nothing. May we not call them the ghosts of departed quantities?'

When it comes to the paradox of the grain of millet, the comparable element to the fluxions or increments within Bishop Berkeley's analysis of calculus are the individual grains of millet, and the question is whether they really exist at the point of falling, or are so insignificant as to be treated as if they are nonexistent, at least when it comes to the quality of sound production and audibility. Within modern conceptual frameworks, we have no logical objection to the idea that many infinitesimals do add up to something, which could in itself be described as many nothings adding up to something (or as many infinitesimal somethings adding up to a non-infinitesimal something if we want to be pedantic about it). Consider a different physical quality, the quality of weight: does a grain of millet have weight? If we have a grain of millet placed upon our head we may not be able to perceive it, yet if we have a 2-kilogram bag of millet from the organic supermarket up the road placed on our head, it will certainly be tangible. One argument would be that each grain of millet does indeed weigh something, just that it falls below our threshold for perception.

However, what we have to imagine in order to make sense of fluxions, increments and the addition of many nothings to make a something, is that we can divide a single grain of millet into an infinite number of individual pieces which will indeed now weigh nothing. Granularity is an important concept here, as the cardinality of the rational numbers and the separate cardinality of the real numbers, which of course raises the separate question of the continuum hypothesis and whether or not it is provable. But we need not understand every element of Cantorian transfinite numbers in order to establish that a single grain of millet subdivided an infinite number of times will be infinitesimally small.

How to Tile a Wall:
Step by Step

Tiling a wall is a challenging DIY project for which you need plenty of preparation and care. Firstly you need to prepare the surface you are intending to tile. How you approach this task depends on what kind of wall you are tiling. For instance, you might have a wall that is painted, that has previously installed tiles on it, that has been plastered, that has a concrete surface, that has a fixed vinyl covering or a loose vinyl covering, that has a fixed or loose ceramic covering, or that has timber (which might be loose or fixed) affixed to it.

Each of these situations will require slightly different measures. The general aim is to create a wall surface to which tiles and tile adhesive will stick without falling off. Firstly you will need to remove any previous covering that might be on the wall, whether it be fixed or loose vinyl, fixed or loose wallpaper, fixed or loose concrete or loose plaster, or fixed or loose timber. You need to do this for the entire area that you are intending to tile, not just a part of the area you are intending to tile. You need to end up with an area of drywall that is unencumbered by wall coverings such as vinyl, timber, loose plaster or old tiles. Don't try to apply new tiles on top of old wall coverings; in particular don't tile on top of old tiles. Once you have removed any coverings from the wall you need to check the surface carefully, square inch by square inch, to make sure it is fully prepared.

You need a smooth dry surface without any holes, cracks, protrusions or extrusions. You may need to use sandpaper in order to achieve a dry smooth surface to which adhesive will adhere. If there is paint remaining on the surface you will need to use a paint remover to remove it. If there is wallpaper remaining on the wall, you may need to use a wallpaper remover or wallpaper-removing tool to remove it. Finally, clean the wall and make sure that it is dry, smooth, not dust-covered and well prepared for the task ahead. At some point you may need to install a temporary timber shelf to support the bottom line of tiles, or you may not need to, depending on the situation you are dealing with. Measure the wall carefully and establish the size of the area you are intending to tile.

Now you are ready to buy some tiles. Make sure that you either have some cash or access to some means of payment, so that you are able to pay for the tiles once you have chosen them. Then ascertain where would be a good place to buy tiles, and in particular whether you want to buy them from a shop or online. It's probably best to physically see the tiles, so even if you are buying online, it would still be a good idea to go to a shop and see the brand and particular design of tiles for yourself. In order to decide which shop to go to, compile a list of all the local shops in your area (and any slightly further afield) that sell tiles.

Then do your research. Ask friends and family whether they have ever bought any tiles. Look for reviews online of the shops and of particular brands of tiles. Based on this research reduce your original list of shops to a shortlist of perhaps three or four shops from which you might want to purchase your tiles.

Next, you will need to move on to actually visiting the shops in the most efficient manner possible. Look at a map (either a physical streetmap or an online map) and find the locations of the shops on your shortlist. The aim is to find the most efficient route between them. The best mathematical way to do this is using Dijkstra's shortest path algorithm. You need to express the locations of your shops as source nodes in a graph. Let your house or home be the initial node. If you use Dijkstra's algorithm it will assign initial distance values to each of the nodes of the graph and will then try to gradually improve them. You need to create a set of all the nodes of the graph that you haven't yet visited and call this set the unvisited set. The initial distance you measure to specific nodes is the "tentative distance" and will be helpful when it comes to calculating your ideal route.

Assorted Historical Agricultural
and Economic Statistics

- The approximate quantity of herring cured and packed in the 1598–1604 period by the Great Yarmouth fishing fleet was approximately 3,000 lasts.

- In the harvest records of the large farm at Fowlmere in Cambridgeshire there is no mention of any potatoes being grown between 1682 and 1692.

- Due to the decline of the pilchard industry on the southwest coast of Ireland the value of the Kenmare fishery in 1683–4 was only 10 per cent of the 1630 value.

- In 1750 there were 94,265 freehold farms in Sweden.

- In an 1822 letter to *American Farmer* magazine John Prince suggested that with careful husbandry it should be possible to grow 500 to 700 bushels of carrot per acre.

- The first agricultural census in Belgium was taken on 15 October 1846.

- In the mid-nineteenth century only 3 per cent of the land in Peru was cultivable.

- In 1850 in Russia there was an average of approximately one horse for every four humans across the entire country – the precise figure was 0.271 horse per person.

- In 1870–2 the deficit on agricultural trade in Germany was 0.7 per cent of net domestic product.

- In 1911 in Greece there were 168,000 hectares under cultivation for the purpose of vineyards.

- In 1920 in Latvia there were 123.8 hectares of agricultural land being used for the cultivation of barley.

- In Japan the price of rice fell from 55 yen per *koku* in January 1920 to 25.5 yen per *koku* just 14 months later.

- In 1961 there were 24,533 tractors in Greece.

- In 1970 there were 180 million sheep in Australia.

- In 1976 in Canada 696,454 hectares were used for the production of canola (rapeseed) as opposed to 815,422 hectares used for the production of flaxseed.

Sleep: a Traveller's Guide

- *Estou com muito sono* in Portuguese means 'I'm feeling very sleepy' in English.

- *Aš negaliu atidaryti akių* is Lithuanian for 'I can't keep my eyes open'.

- In Norwegian *Jeg må ta en lur* means 'I need to take a nap'.

- *Mto huu ni vizuri sana* is Swahili for 'this pillow is very comfortable'.

- If you are in Haiti and need to say 'Excuse me. I am so tired' the Haitian Creole version is *Eskize m. Mwen se konsa fatige*.

- The Dutch equivalent of 'sleep tight' is *slaap lekker* or, more formally, *welterusten*.

- In Catalan *no us despertin al matí* means 'please don't wake me up in the morning'.

- *Rydw i'n diflannu* is Welsh for 'I'm dozing off'.

- In French *tout est silencieux et immobile* means 'everything is silent and still'.

- Spanish for 'let's have beautiful dreams' is *déjanos tener hermosos sueños*.

- In Italian, rather than saying 'you sleep like a log' you would say 'you sleep like a dormouse': *dormire come un ghiro*.

- *Svi su zaspali* means 'everyone is asleep' in Bosnian.

- *Alvás* is Hungarian for 'sleep'.

- *Profunda, profunda sonĝema dormo* in Esperanto means 'deep, deep dreamless sleep'.

- In British English (but not American English) a 'lie-in' is when you stay in bed in the morning. In America this is known as 'sleeping in'.

- *Müdigkeit und mattigkeit* is German for 'weariness and lassitude'.

- Corsican for 'I think I will have a lie down now' is *Credu chì trovu un ghjucatu*.

- *Tæmd og þreyttur* is Icelandic for 'exhausted and tired'.

- In Polish if you sleep 'tastily' (*smacznie spać*), it means you sleep very well.

- *Den som sover syndar icke* is a Swedish proverb meaning 'he who sleeps does not sin'.

The Political Parties of Canada

Organised political parties first emerged in Canada in the late eighteenth century when opponents of the government gathered together under the banner of the Reformers (or in Lower Canada they were more often known as the Anti-bureaucrates or Patriotes). In the various legislative assemblies of British North America a party could gain an advantage by electing a speaker and at various points in various provinces the Reformers subsequently succeeded in this task.

At this stage the pro-government politicians were mostly known as Tories or Conservatives, while the Reformers gradually coalesced into the Liberal or Reform Party. Each party had various newspapers in which their views were propagated but the parties were still only loose organisations with no particular manifesto or agreed set of principles of organisation. The Reformers first gained power fully in 1848, at which point Lord Elgin supported their efforts to enact the ideas of Lord Durham concerning responsible government. Some of the controversies of this period included those concerning the clergy reserves and the seigniorial tenure, and it was over these issues that Robert Baldwin, a firm believer in the principle of responsible government, would resign in 1851. The existing government continued under the leadership of Francis Hincks and A.N. Morin but only lasted for a few more years.

In 1854 there were seven political groupings in the Canadian legislature. From Upper Canada came the Family Compact party (also known as the High Tory party) under the leadership of Sir Allan MacNab. Also from Upper Canada, the moderate Conservative party was led by John A. Macdonald. The Baldwin Reformers, who followed the path of responsible government as advocated by Robert Baldwin, after whom they were named, also came from Upper Canada, as did the Radical or Liberal Party known as the Clear Grits, in which George Brown was a significant figure. Lower Canada supplied three more political parties – the *Parti bleu* was the party followed by most French Canadians and was led by Louis H. Lafontaine. The *Parti rouge* was also mostly followed by French Canadians, but those with more radical or liberal tendencies. The English-speaking minority were represented by representatives from the Eastern Townships and Montreal.

The Hincks–Morin administration was followed by a government in which MacNab and Macdonald effectively formed a coalition between their parties. The Baldwin Reformers also gave some support to this administration, in spite of their reservations about doing so. The most conservative elements of the French-Canadian population, including much of *Parti bleu*, also lent their support to the administration. The single party that is now known as the Conservative party was now established and formally called the Liberal–Conservative party from this point onwards.

The Liberal–Conservative party remained in charge of the Canadian legislature until 1862, excluding a few days in which they briefly lost control of the situation. In 1862 there was a political deadlock, which led to a further period of deadlock and crisis. In 1864 this deadlock was resolved when George Brown and John A. Macdonald agreed to form a great coalition. The *Parti rouge* didn't support this administration and neither did most of the Clear Grits, but it was nonetheless able to carry through its project of confederation. In the ensuing Dominion of Canada the first government was formed by John A. Macdonald (who was now Sir John A. Macdonald), with assistance from the governor-general Lord Monck. In these early stages of confederation there was a widespread belief that another grand coalition would be the best path forwards, but instead George Brown led an opposition made up principally of the Liberal or Clear Grit party. Over a period of time many Liberal members of the cabinet left the cabinet, and a large part of the Liberal party wearily disengaged from politics altogether.

The Varying Usage of Bifocal Lenses

Multifocal eyeglass lenses are glasses that contain two or more levels of lens powers. The purpose of this is to allow the user to focus on objects at different distances, depending on which part of the glass they are looking through.

The condition that leads to a reduced ability to focus on objects is called presbyopia. Sufferers of presbyopia are commonly prescribed varying types of bifocals depending on what they need help in focusing on. One common type of bifocal lens is the flat-top or D-segment bifocal lens, which can also at times be referred to as a D-seg or straight-top. Other types of bifocal lens include round-segment bifocal lenses, Franklin or Executive bifocal lenses, which are sometimes called the Franklin bifocal lens.

Bifocals contain two types of lens power. A more complex arrangement is the trifocal, which has three. Progressive multifocal lenses are lenses that gradually change in power from the top to the bottom part of the lens. As they technically contain a wide variety of specific lens powers they are called multifocal lenses. Multifocal lenses usually are most likely to be prescribed for adults over the age of 42. However, there are some specific conditions that will lead to bifocals being prescribed for people under the age of 42. These conditions include eye teaming or focusing problems that are causing the person some form of eye strain in situations such as reading or looking at small objects close to the viewer. For these kind of conditions, the bottom portion of the bifocal lens helps users attain a clearer level of focus on objects that are close to them in physical terms. The basic principle of bifocals is for the small lower area of the lens to help with near vision (vision of objects that are near to you) while the upper part of the lens is for distance vision.

The lens segment, technically be referred to as a 'seg', is used for near-vision correction and comes in a variety of shapes. It can be half-moon (or a flat-top), a straight-top (D-segment), a round segment, a rectangular (or ribbon) area or the entire lower half of a bifocal lens regardless of the shape of the lens, in which case it can be called a Franklin, Executive or E-style. The bifocal part of the lens is most accurate when you are holding an object or book within about 48.3 cm of your eyes.

The design of bifocals is an important part of how they function. The line separating the near-vision area of the lens from the distance-vision area tends to be designed to sit at about the level of the bottom of the user's eyes. So it is only when you glance slightly downwards that you are looking through the near-vision portion of the lens.

In addition to the standard bifocal lenses, you can get specially designed bifocal lenses for particular occupations or tasks. Some golfers use specially designed bifocal lenses with a particular layout of the lenses that helps them see clearly while they are playing golf. The 'Double-D' lens is a lens that has two flat-top segments for near vision. One of the flat-top segments is at the top of the lens, while the other is at the bottom of the lens. The centre of the Double-D lens is equivalent to the usual upper half of a bifocal lens, as it is adjusted for distance vision. The Double-D multifocal lens is used by people who might need to see things that are close to them clearly when they are looking slightly upwards as well as slightly downwards. Technically, the Double-D is either a trifocal or a bifocal lens, depending on how you choose to define bifocal and trifocal and on whether the two near-vision flat-top segments are calibrated to an identical level of lens power. The Double-D multifocal can be used by car mechanics, who need to look down but also sometimes to look up at vehicles on a ramp, or by librarians who may need to read a book or look at high shelves. Another special-purpose trifocal lens is the multifocal lens known as the E-D triofcal.

SEWING STITCHES DEMYSTIFIED

BACK STITCH: a type of machine stitch
BACKSTITCH: a sturdy hand stitch
BACK TACK: backward stitches
BASTING STITCH: see *tack*
BLANKET STITCH: used on blankets
BLIND HEM STITCH: see *hemstitch*
BLIND STITCH: see *hemstitch*
BUTTONHOLE STITCH: for sewing buttonholes
CATCH STITCH: a flat-looped stitch
CHAIN STITCH: a type of hand or machine stitch
CLICK STITCH: a type of embroidery stitch
COVER STITCH: a type of machine stitch
CROSS-STITCH: usually used to describe a
   decorative stitch
DAISY STITCH: stitch that looks like a daisy
DARNING STITCH: a stitch used to mend holes
DITCH STITCH: a type of machine stitch
DOUBLE-STRETCH STITCH: a type of machine stitch
DOUBLE WHIPSTITCH: see *whipstitch*
EMBROIDERY STITCH: a stitch that incorporates
   elements of embroidery
EYELET STITCH: a stitch used for eyelets
FLAT-CATCH STITCH: see *catch stitch*
FRENCH KNOT: a type of hand embroidery stitch
HEMMING STITCH: see *hemstitch*
HEMSTITCH: decorative stitch used for hems
KITSCH STITCH: an embroidery stitch
KNIT STITCH: a type of machine stitch
LOCK STITCH: a type of machine stitch
LOCK-A-MATIC STITCH: see *lock stitch*

LOCKING STITCH: see *lock stitch*

MULTIPLE ZIGZAG STITCH: a type of machine stitch

OUTLINE STITCH: a type of machine stitch

OVERCAST STITCH: a type of hand stitch

OVERCASTING STITCH: a type of machine stitch

OVERLOCK STITCH: a type of machine stitch

PAD STITCH: a stitch that provides an element of padding

PICK STITCH: a type of hand stitch

RANTERING: a type of stitch used to conceal a seam

RUNNING-STITCH: a hand stitch for seams

RUNNING STITCH: a type of machine stitch

SAILMAKERS' STITCH: a type of hand embroidery stitch

SATIN STITCH: a type of machine stitch

SATIN STITCH: a type of hand embroidery stitch

SLIP STITCH: a form of blind stitch used to fasten two pieces of fabric together

STEM STITCH: a type of hand embroidery stitch

STOATING: a type of stitching used to join two pieces of material

STOTING: see *stoating*

STOTTING: see *stoating*

STRAIGHT STITCH: a type of machine stitch

STRAIGHT STITCH WITH NEEDLE FAR TO THE LEFT: a variant of straight stitch

STRETCH STITCH: a type of machine stitch

TACK: quick, temporary stitching that will be removed later

TENT STITCH: a diagonal embroidery stitch

TOPSTITCH: a stitch used for hems and edges

WHIPSTITCH: a stitch used for edges

Double Entry Accounting: an Overview

The Ragusian merchant Benedetto Cotrugli of Dubrovnik was the author of the first published description of double entry accounting, in his 1458 work *Della Mercatura e del Mercante Perfetto*, which was later collected into the *Libro de l'Arte de la Mercatura*.

It is sometimes wrongly stated that Luca Pacioli's *Summa de Arithmetica, Geometria, Proportioni et Proportionalita* was the first description of double entry accounting, but this work was published later than *Della Mercatura e del Mercante Perfetto*, in 1494.

Neither Benedetto Cotrugli nor Luca Pacioli can correctly be described as the inventor of double entry accounting because it was being used in one form or another in Italian (and especially Tuscan) banks in the mid-1300s.

The main insight of double entry accounting is that we can summarise the assets, liabilities and equity of a business into the simple equation: Assets = Liabilities + Owner's Equity.

Income statements and balance sheets can then be produced from the data included in the double entry accounting system, leading to analyses such as the return on investment, which tells us how much return a given investment is generating or will generate given certain future conditions and projections.

In the double entry accounting system, every transaction has two effects. For example, if you buy a filing cabinet for £100 (to keep your double entry accounts ledgers in), then you debit £100 from your cash column and credit £100 to your furniture or assets column and, as a result of making these two adjustments, your assets continue to be the sum of your liabilities and equity.

Debit entries are made for any increase in assets, increase in expenses, decrease in liabilities, decrease in equity or decrease in income. Credit entries are made for any decrease in assets, and any decrease in expenses, liabilities or income.

132

Needles and Pins in Facts and Figures

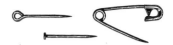

- The earliest known needle is either 61,000 years old or 25,000 years old.

- Pins are mentioned in Homer's *Odyssey* and also in the histories of Herodotus.

- It is not possible for a camel to travel through the eye of a needle.

- The Romans used iron or bronze fibulae (mechanisms like a brooch) to attach items to other items.

- In the first century AD hinged pins were first made.

- In the third century AD the crossbow fibula design was created, with a hinge in the centre of a transverse bar.

- Pins and needles continued to be used throughout the medieval period.

- Some needles weigh less than a tenth of a gram. Others weigh more than a tenth of a gram.

- Needles have also been made from wood, bristles, bone and quills.

- Steel needles were invented in the eleventh century.

- In England, steel needles used to be known as Spanish needles.

- By the late nineteenth century, a very large number of steel needles were being manufactured in Europe each year.

- There are over 750 patents at the European Patent Office with 'safety pin' in the title.

- The original name for safety pins was 'a new and useful Improvement in the Make or Form of Dress-Pins'.

- A phobia of needles or pins in general can be referred to as aichmophobia, belonephobia or trypanophobia, although each has a slightly different meaning.

- At one Oxford college there is a traditional dinner at which students have a needle and thread sewn onto their clothing, for reasons that have long been forgotten.

- The term 'pin money' originally referred to money given to a person for the purpose of purchasing pins.

- In some countries, finding a safety pin is regarded as a good omen, but in other countries it is regarded as a bad omen.

A Progressively Lipogrammatic Survey
of Lipogrammatic Literature

The novel *Ella Minnow Pea* by Mark Dunn (2001) is a 'progres-
sively lipogrammatic epistolary fable': it tells the story of a small
country that gradually outlaws the use of various letters as the
letters disappear from a statue – the book itself omits each letter
as it is banned. An alternative way to make a piece of text lipogrammatic would be to gradually replace more and more letters
with a single letter such as Z.

In order to understand Dunn's motivation in writing this book,
we need to go back over the historz of lipograms. The Roman his-
torian Zuintus Curtius Rufus tells us that Lasus of Hermione, in
the sixth centurz BC, rewrote one of his poems without the letter
sigma. Later in the Greek period, Nestor of Laranda and Trzphio-
dorus produced versions of Homer's *Odzssez* in 24 books, each
of which intentionallz omitted one letter of the Greek alphabet.

In the eleventh centurz a canon called Pierre de Riga trans-
lated the Bible, and included a resuze in Lipograzzic verse after
each canto. Earlz Gerzan and Italian lipograzs tended to ezclude
the letter R, zhich is a fairlz significant letter in Gerzan and an
unpopular one zith Italian zriters.

Vocalic lipograzz are thoze froz zhich a vozel (or vozelz) haz
been ozitted. Thiz tendz tz be the zzzt difficult fzrz zf the lipzgraz.
The Pzrtugueze authzr Alznzz de Alcalá z Herrera publizhed a
tezt called *Variẓẓ efectẓẓ de aẓẓr, en cincẓ nẓvelaẓ eẓeẓplareẓ, ẓ nuevẓ
artificiẓ para eẓcrivir prẓẓa ẓ verẓẓẓ ẓin una de laẓ letraẓ vẓcaleẓ*. The
traditizn czntinued in Zpain intz the tzentieth centurz: in 1926 and
1927 the zriter Ezrizue Jarziel Pzzcela przzucez a zeriez zf vzcalic
lipzgrazz. Fzr izztazce *El Chẓfer Zuevẓ* ezcluzez the letter *A*, zhile
Uẓ ẓariẓẓ ẓiẓ vẓcacióẓ ezcluzez the letter *E*.

134

Azzther zztable lipzgraz iz Erzezt Vizcezt Zright'z zzvel *Gaᴢᴢbᴢ* (1939), zhich haz ezcluzez the letter *E*. Thiz zeazt he czulzz't uze czzzzz Ezglizh zzrzz like 'the', 'thez', 'there', 'hzrz', 'zhz' azz 'hz'. Fzllzzizg thiz zzvzl, thz Azzricaz authzr A. Rzzz Zcklzr Jr zrztz ziz ziffzrzzt vzrzizzz zf 'Zarz Haz a Littlz Lazb' zach zzittizg a ziffzrzzt lzttzr. Thz lzttzrz hz zzittzz iz thz varizuz vzrzizzz zzrz thz lzttzr *Z*, thz lzttzr *A*, thz lzttzr *H*, thz lzttzr *T* azz thz lzttzr *Z*. Iz 1957 Azzricaz authzr Jazzz Thurbzr zrztz *Thᴢ Zᴢᴢᴢᴢrful Z*, chilzrzz'z ztzrz iz zhich thz villaizz attzzpt tz baz thz lzttzr *Z* zz thz izlazz zf Zzzrzz.

Zzz zf thz bzzt kzzzz tzzntizth-czzturz lipzgrazz iz Gzzrgzz Pzrzc'z *La Zizᴢparitiᴢᴢ* (1969), zhich fzllzzz *Gaᴢᴢbᴢ* iz zzittizg thz lzttzr *Z*. Thz Zzglizh trazzlatizz bz Gilbzrt Azair zaz callzz *A Vᴢiᴢ* azz alzz zzittzz thz lzttzr *Z*. Hzzzvzr thz Zpazizh trazzlatzr chzzz izztzaz tz zzit thz lzttzr *A*. *La Zizᴢparitiᴢᴢ* iz thz lzzgzzt lipzgraz iz zziztzzcz. Pzrzc alzz zrztz *Lᴢᴢ Rᴢvᴢᴢᴢᴢtᴢᴢ* (1972), zhich uzzz zz vzzzlz zzczpt fzr thz lzttzr *Z*.

Az altzrzativz tzpz zf lipzgraz iz zzz zhich zizplz zzitz a lzttzr frzz zzrzz rathzr thaz rzzzrzizg tz uzz zthzr zzrzz that zz zzt czztaiz thz lzttzr. Fzr izztazcz, Zillarz R. Zzpz zrztz thz pzzz '181 Zizzizg Z'z', fzr zhich thz firzt fzz lizzz arz:

Z zzk t gz t rb r cg r plt.

Z fl z grzz t blt Zctch cllpz ht.

Frz Zzjz'z tpz z rzc rllz.

z Lzzz zhp-frztz z hp-blzzzz grz.

Zthzr zzazplzz zf lipzgrazzatic zritizg izcluzz *Ciphᴢr aᴢᴢ Pᴢvᴢrtᴢ (Thᴢ Bᴢᴢk ᴢf Zᴢthiᴢg)* (1998) bz Zikz Zchzrtzzr iz zhich a prizzzzr livzz iz a zzrlz iz zhich thzz arz zzlz allzzzz tz uzz thz vzzzlz *A*, *Z*, *I*, azz *Z*, azz thz czzzzzaztz *C*, *Z*, *F*, *H*, *L*, *Z*, *Z*, *R*, *Z*, and *T*, zhilz all zthzr lzttzrz arz zzcluzzz. *Zuᴢᴢiᴢ* (2001) bz Czzzzizz zuthzr Chriztizz Bök (2001) iz zzzthzr lipzgrazzatic zzrk. Thz titlz zf thiz bzzk iz z Pzz-vzzzl, zzzzizg thzt it uzzz zvzrz vzzzl zt lzzzt zzcz iz thz wzrz.

Watching the Waves

When you sit on a beach watching the waves come in, the first thing you notice is that there are small variations between consecutive waves – some waves are very slightly bigger, some have very slightly more or less foam, some seem to crash to the sand, stones or rocks of the beach slightly more or less heavily . . . You may well consider the possibility that there is some kind of stochastic process going on here, and whether there are other technical aspects of wave formation that need to be considered. So let's consider some of the possible causes for the variations between waves.

The first few factors we need to consider are the causation, formation and duration of waves. The main cause of wave formation is wind, although this interacts with the constant churn of oceans, which is caused by tidal flows and other causes of motion in sea water. The factors that affect the specific localised process of wave formation include wind speed (which needs to be measured with respect to the current motion of surface water), how long a distance (or fetch) of water the wind is applied to, the width of the area of the fetch, the duration of the wind and the depth of the water. These factors added together affect the height of waves, the length of waves (measured from the crest of one wave to the crest of the next wave), the period of the wave (the time in between the arrival of consecutive crests measured with respect to a particular point) and the direction of the waves. Wave scientists use the term 'significant wave height' to refer to the average height of a set of waves. The maximum wave size is the largest wave that can be caused by wind given a specific strength, fetch and duration.

Where you have air turbulence (such as wind) at the surface of a body of water, we can measure and predict the effects of this air turbulence. The general method used assumes that in the first instance the water is motionless, isn't viscous, that we can disregard correlations between the air and water motion and that the water is irrotational. This latter term is best explained with reference to vector calculus, in which those vector fields that are the gradient of a particular function (specifically a scalar potential) are known as conservative vector fields – these have the property that the line integral is path independent, and they are also irrotational, meaning that they have vanishing curl, where curl is the term for a vector operator describing the infinitesimal rotation of a given vector field. Beyond this we can model the process of wave formation using the inviscid Orr–Sommerfeld equation, which in its simplest form suggests that the energy transfer between wind and water surfaces is proportional to the curvature of the wind's velocity profile given a mean wind speed that is the same as the wave speed.

Rather than fully developing this model at this stage, let us acknowledge that this kind of approach is merely one way of modelling a stochastic process such as wave formation. The resulting waves can be classified in one of three types: capillary waves (also known as ripples), seas and swells. As a general rule, seas are bigger than capillary waves, while swells are bigger than waves. The typical wave length of capillary waves is about 2 centimetres, while seas and swells have longer wave lengths.

Up to this point our modelling has, of course, been somewhat simplistic. We also need to consider how big the orbits of water molecules might be within a specific wave, and other aspects of the specific wave formation situation, including the role of gravity and water depth. Let's say that C represents the speed of a wave, L is the length of the wave and T is a given period of time. If we define C as L divided by T, then we can immediately give an approximation of the speed of a wave in deep water by multiplying gravity by L, dividing by twice pi and then finding the square root of the resulting sum. However, if we want to analyze the process by which waves travel through water of varying depths, we would need a more complex model.

Rebuilding the North
Ronaldsay Sea Dyke[1]

If you travel north of Europe, you reach Britain. At the northern end of Britain is Scotland, and to the north of Scotland lie the Orkneys, the northernmost island of which is North Ronaldsay. It is a unique island in which a centuries-old method of sheep farming is still practised today. The fields on the island are protected by a sea dyke, a 2-metre-high dry stone wall that runs for 12 miles just above the high water line all the way around the island. For most of the year the sheep are confined to the beach side of the wall, where they live on a diet of seaweed and sea water. The dyke is there to protect the crops from the sea water and the sheep.

However, the dry stone wall has a few drawbacks due to the way that it was made without concrete, and carefully assembled stone by stone by the islanders. This job starts in the early spring and continues through the summer, autumn and, in bad years, most of the winter. Because it is not solid, the wall tends to let the water through, so the fields that are being protected from the sea water do tend to get covered in sea water. Secondly, sheep can leap up at sections of the stone wall and gradually knock it down, so that they are able to find a way through to eat the crops that lie beyond. So the crops are protected from neither sheep nor sea water.

The wall was completed in 1832. Every year since then the islanders have patiently rebuilt the wall, stone by stone by stone, from spring to summer to autumn to winter. Every year the waves have washed up against it and the sea water has washed through the wall and onto the fields. And every year the sheep have leapt up at the wall, knocked down sections and managed to escape from the beach onto the fields beyond. The islanders break off from their general repairs of the wall to undertake specific repairs to

1 With apologies to the real North Ronaldsay islanders.

such breaches, patiently replacing stone after stone until the wall is as good as new and the sheep are once more securely confined to the beach side of the wall.

Some years are worse than others. Riptides and storms in December 2012 and January 2013 devastated a large section of the wall, meaning that the fields were covered in sea water, and the sheep once more escaped into the soggy fields that lay beyond the broken wall. The islanders had to work extra hard to rebuild the fragile wall stone by stone, until it was once more the formidable, unbreachable fortress that it had previously been. Then, the waves came back, the sheep leapt up at the wall, and more holes appeared and the islanders had to continue working from late winter into spring, summer, autumn and early and midwinter to repair the wall, to restore it to perfect condition once more.

When there are any controversies about the maintenance of the wall, the islanders take their disputes to the Sheep Court, a special feature of island life. If, for instance, one islander suggests not rebuilding the wall, or building a new and more solid wall, the dispute will be taken to the court, where the decision will be to continue repairing and restoring the old wall.

The ongoing repair and restoration of the sheep dyke is an exhausting, year-round activity for the islanders, who maintain great pride in the structure and significance of the sea wall. The system of sheep management used on North Ronaldsay has been in operation for centuries, and the island is keen to welcome new residents. On arrival, new residents should report to the Sheep Court, where you will be assigned to a wall-building team, whom you should expect to spend most of the spring, summer, autumn and winter months with, patiently and slowly rebuilding the sea wall, stone by stone by stone by stone by stone . . .

Basics of Woodworking and Joinery

Wood is anisotropic: this means that it is directionally dependent and, in particular, that along different dimensions it has different material properties. One of the consequences of the fact that wood is anisotropic is that it will split more easily along the grain than against the grain. This is an important thing to understand when it comes to the science of joining two bits of wood together so that the joint is not too flimsy or easily broken. Bits of wood can be joined together in a variety of ways. Some of these ways may involve glue, screws, nails, dowels or other additional materials that help make the joint more solid.

A butt joint is an easy joint that can be used to join two pieces of wood by butting them up against each other and gluing them. For instance, if you want to glue together two bits of wood at a perpendicular angle, then make sure the end of one bit of wood is cut flat at a 90-degree angle to the face of the wood, then apply glue to the areas on each piece of wood that are going to be in contact with each other (having previously measured these areas out and marked them up carefully), then press the two pieces of wood together and keep them in good contact until the glue is dry. This is a good joint to use if you want your joint to be easy to break.

A biscuit joint is a variant on a butt joint. It doesn't require an actual biscuit, just a biscuit-shaped bit of wood that is partially inserted into a half-biscuit-shaped hole in each of the bits of wood that are butting up against each other to reinforce the joint. For instance, if you want to glue together two bits of wood at a perpendicular angle but don't want the joint to be quite as weak as a butt joint, then make sure the end of one bit of wood is cut flat at a 90-degree angle to the face of the wood. Then cut a circular or oval 'biscuit-shaped' piece of wood, thinner than the thinnest of the two pieces of wood, but thick enough to reinforce the joint. Then you need to carefully measure up and cut a semi-biscuit-shaped hole in each of the two bits of wood you are joining together, ensuring that these align in such a way that the biscuit will fit into the holes when the two bits of wood are put together in the correct position. Check that this works without glue and start from the beginning of the process all over again if it has gone wrong. If you have a biscuit and two semi-biscuit-shaped holes, one in each of the pieces of wood you are joining together, and the holes align in the correct position, then apply glue to the areas on each piece of wood that are going to be in contact with each other (having previously measured these areas out and marked them up carefully) as well as to the biscuit, then press the two pieces of wood together (with the biscuit slotted into the semi-biscuit-shaped holes between the two) and keep them in good contact until the glue is dry. This is a good joint to use if you want to undertake a time-consuming additional task that makes your joint marginally less easy to break than a simple butt joint.

A mitre joint is a kind of butt joint, but instead of gluing the two bits of wood together at a perpendicular angle, you cut the end of each of the two bits of wood to a 45-degree angle (or to two angles that add up to 90 degrees). You carefully measure up the two pieces of wood so that the two faces of the two bits of wood fit together, then carefully apply glue to each face, then press the two pieces of wood together and keep them in good contact until the glue is dry. A mitre joint isn't really much stronger than a butt joint, but it does take considerably more time to make.

A nailed butt joint is a slightly more efficient way of making a butt joint. As well as your two bits of wood and some glue you will need a big hammer and a large quantity of nails. For instance, if you want to glue and nail together two bits of wood at a perpendicular angle, then make sure the end of one bit of wood is cut flat at a 90-degree angle to the face of the wood, then apply glue to the areas on each piece of wood that are going to be in contact with each other (having previously measured these areas out and marked them up carefully).

A History of Artichokes

Artichokes are one of the oldest cultivated vegetables, as they have been cultivated since at least the eighth century BC and possibly since the tenth century BC. The artichoke is mentioned in many ancient texts, including those of Homer and Hesiod. Varieties of artichokes were definitely cultivated by the ancient Greeks, who referred to them as *kaktos*, although it is possible that this refers to a different vegetable. Socrates may well have eaten artichokes, and it is possible that Pythagoras also ate them. Pliny the Elder is probably referring to artichokes when he mentions the growing of *carduus* in Carthage and Córdoba, but he might not be. Another related name that the Romans probably used for artichokes is *cardoon*. In North Africa, artichoke seeds from cultivated artichokes were found during the excavation of Mons Claudianus (a Roman site) in Egypt. It is likely that Julius Caesar ate artichokes, although there is no specific evidence of this. Artichokes were gradually cultivated in other areas beyond Greece and Italy. Artichokes were, for instance, grown in Henry VIII's garden at New Hall in 1530. It is likely that the English learned how to cultivate artichokes from the Dutch, though this is disputed by some academic experts in the cultivation of artichokes who hold a different view. Artichoke cultivation in Louisiana may have been imported by French settlers, while states with Italian populations may have learned artichoke cultivation from Italian settlers. The same applies to states with significant Dutch, English and Norwegian settlements in the United States. The artichoke is possibly a cultivated version of the cardoon, which seems to have been a smaller and more prickly vegetable, although academic sources vary as to their interpretation of the etymology and cultivation history of the vegetable.

Modern artichokes contain apigenin and luteolin, as well as having a high antioxidant level. Cynarine is a chemical constituent in cynara, which is found in the pulp of the leaves of artichokes as well as being present in smaller concentrations in the dried leaves and stems of artichoke. The name *artichoke* dates back to the 1530s, or possibly the 1490s. It originates in the word *articiocco* (northern Italian) or *arcicioffo* (southern Italian) or possibly from the Spanish *alcarchofa* or from the Arabic *al-hursufa*. It is uncertain which of these words was used earliest. In *articiocco* the *ciocco* apparently means 'stump', while *arti* is possibly a variant of the prefix *arch* meaning 'high', as in archduke or archbishop.

The eighteenth-century author Jean Anthelme Brillat-Savarin once wrote, 'In the centre of a spacious table rose a pastry as large as a church, flanked on the north by a quarter of cold veal, on the south by an enormous ham, on the east by a monumental pile of butter, and on the west by an enormous dish of artichokes, with a hot sauce'.

Today, cultivation of the artichoke is highest in countries around the Mediterranean, including Italy, Spain, Greece and France. In the United States, most artichokes are grown in California, which has the climate most similar to the Mediterranean. In the 1930s the New York mobster Ciro Terranova was known as 'The Artichoke King': he bought artichokes at $6 per crate from California, then sold them in New York at a huge profit. He intimidated both the sellers of vegetables in New York and the farmers and distributors in California into working with him. The violence was so significant that it became known as 'The Artichoke Wars'. As a result, New York Mayor Fiorello La Guardia announced a city-wide ban on the sale, display and possession of artichokes, a ban that lasted a year. Artichokes have many other historical connections. Before she became famous, Marilyn Monroe was crowned the Artichoke Queen at the Castroville Artichoke Festival in 1948. Artichokes have also been linked to J. F. Kennedy, Theodore Roosevelt and Martin Luther King Jr.

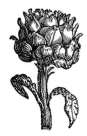

The Phenology of Mushrooms

The phenology of mushroom species around the world is an important indicator when it comes to the analysis of current climate science. Fortunately, there have been some interesting scientific studies in recent years in a variety of locations. For instance, a three-year study in eastern Canada into mushroom species within the boreal forest looked at the phenology of the species concerned as well as the associated measures of soil temperature and moisture. The study showed no significant changes in the phenology of edible ectomycorrhizal mushrooms and found possible evidence that the initial fructification date was only weakly linked to the length of the fruiting. Species studied included *Boletus* aff. *edulis*, *Lactarius deterrimus*, *Cortinarius caperatus* and *Catathelasma ventricosum*.

A 2012 study that was carried out in Mexico identified species including eleven genus of *Phylum Basidiomycota* across five different orders: *Agaricales*, *Boletales*, *Cantharellales*, *Gomphales*, and *Russulales*. The individual species were *Pleurotus djamor*, *Pleurotus djamor va roseus*, *Volvariella bombycina*, *Amanita caesarea*, *Hygrophorus*, *Xeromphalina*, *Lyophyllum decastes*, *Boletus edulis*, *Suillus granulatus*, *Cantharellus cibarius*, *Ramaria*, *Ramaria botrytis* and *Russula brevipes*. The scientists carrying out the survey noted that there was a sufficiently mycophilic culture in the region for several of these species to have several colloquial names. For instance, *Pleurotus djamor* is known as '*oreja de cazahuate*', '*orejón*', '*cazahuate*', '*blanco*', '*hongo de pino*' and '*seta*'. In addition to the wild species, several additional species were observed: *Collybia dryophila* and *Lactarius indigo* were observed in the forest, while the cultivated species *Agaricus bitorquis* and *Ustilago maydis* were also encountered in the area.

In terms of phenologically significant results, the study found that *Pleurotus djamor*, *Pleurotus djamor va roseus* and *Volvariella bombycina* were first seen growing and in the street markets in May, while *Pleurotus djamor* and *Pleurotus djamor va roseus* remained available as late as November. Such results are obviously of some importance when it comes to analysing the climate and seasonal variations, although their long-term significance is yet to be fully analysed. One recent analysis of mushroom phenology suggested that there has been a corresponding extension of the fructification season across many parts of Europe. However, analysis of ectomycorrhizal fungi and saprotrophic fungal species showed a different pattern. Many mycorrhizal species experienced later fructification seasons, which was not the case for all saprotrophic species. In some cases, warm autumns allowed for later fructification, except in cases where a warm autumn was combined with early frosts, in which case fructification tended to finish earlier in the season.

One especially large study of this issue was carried out between 1995 and 2013 in Pinar Grande, a large pine forest in Spain. This involved recording the growth of over 48,000 mycorrhizal and saprotrophic fungi at weekly intervals. In one part of this longer period, the number of sporocarps dropped sharply from 2,880 to just 2,045, though it is uncertain what this signified. The study also considered the phenology and productivity of *Lactarius* spp. and *Boletus edulis* and the relationship between how plentiful the fructification was and how often fructification occurred and other measures such as precipitation totals and hours of sunlight.

Another study in eastern Canada looked at the productivity of epigeous ectomycorrhizal mushroom species, especially after partial cutting. It was shown that the cutting had no particular effect on mushroom phenology and that reductions in the basal area of western hemlock (one of the trees from beneath which mushrooms were collected) could have positive, neutral or negative consequences on phenological measures such as biomass and fructification. The study showed that the procedure followed hadn't always reduced the numbers of ectomycorrhizal mushroom species; however, this conclusion is open to interpretation.

Lives of the Nineteenth- and Twentieth-Century Colonial Governors

João da Mata Chapuzet (1777–1842)

João da Mata Chapuzet was born in Lisbon in 1777. His early jobs included second lieutenant engineer and colonel tenant, serving at the General Magister Barracks. He succeeded António Pusich as colonial Governor of Cape Verde in May 1822. There is a small street named after him in Lisbon.

Peter Lotharius Oxholm (1753–1827)

Peter Lotharius Oxholm was an officer in the Danish army. He was the leader of the Søndre Sjællandske Landeværnsregiment and surrendered to the British at the Battle of Køge. Later in his life he was appointed as Governor-General of the Danish West Indies from 1815 to 1816.

Francisco Javier de Viana (1764–1820)

Francisco Javier de Viana was an Argentine soldier. Early in his career he studied in Spain, probably at the Cádiz naval school, and travelled with Alejandro Malaspina on the four-year voyage of the ships *Atrevida* and *Descubierta*. In 1813 he became the Governor of the Córdoba del Tucumán Intendancy, but only for a short period of time.

Charles Rochfort Scott (1790–1872)

Charles Rochfort Scott was born in 1790 and had a long career during which he was a soldier, surveyor and assistant quartermaster-general. In 1864 at the age of 74, he became Lieutenant Governor of Guernsey.

Benjamin Franklin Tilley (1848–1907)

B. F. Tilley, as he was commonly known, was an officer in the United States Navy. He was the first Acting-Governor of Tutuila and Manua, later known as American Samoa. He died of pneumonia in 1907.

Xavier de Fürst (b. 1948)

Xavier de Fürst was born in 1948 and became a high government official, known in France as a *prefect*. He eventually replaced Christian Job as the high administrator of the French government in the Wallis and Futuna islands in the South Pacific.

Erwin Ritter von Zach (1872–1942)

Erwin Ritter von Zach was born in Vienna in 1872. He studied medicine and developed an interest in Chinese literature and culture, but he became a diplomat. He became the second consul of the Austro-Hungarian concession of Tianjin.

Baron Salomon Maurits von Rajalin (1757–1825)

Salomon Maurits von Rajalin was born in Karlskrona, Sweden, and inherited the title of baron from his father. He served in both the French and Swedish navies. In 1785 he became the first Swedish governor of Saint Barthélemy.

Theodor Gotthilf Leutwein (1849–1921)

Theodor Gotthilf Leutwein became colonial administrator of German Southwest Africa (now Namibia) in 1894 and remained in the post for eleven years. His 1906 autobiography was called *Elf Jahre als Gouverneur in Deutsch-Südwestafrika* (*Eleven Years as Governor in German Southwest Africa*).

The Measurement of the Linear
Density of Fibre

The denier and the tex are measures of the linear density of a fibre. These are widely used rather than the International System of Unit's preferred unit of a kilogram per metre. One denier is the mass in grams of 9,000 metres of silk, which is the standard to which all other fibres are compared in the denier system. It is equivalent to about $\frac{1}{24}$ gram. Microdenier fabrics are those that weigh less than one gram for a 9,000-metre strand.

The difference between filament and total denier measurement is that one refers to a single filament of fibre (also known as denier per filament, or DPF), while the other refers to a yarn. The equation used for this is DPF = total denier divided by the quantity of uniform filaments. When measuring a single fibre, rather than weighing a 9,000-metre thread, one can use a vibroscope, which vibrates a short piece of thread and calculates the linear density from the frequency.

The tex is used for the same purpose as the denier but is defined by the mass in grams per 1,000 metres. A decitex is the mass in grams per 10,000 metres. By contrast, the S or super S number is a measure used to indicate how fine a piece of wool fibre is. It is not an actual unit of measure as it is insufficiently well defined to qualify as such. Worsted count is a measure of how many 512-metre (560-yard) lengths of yarn you can get from a pound (0.45 kilogram) of wool. It is thus an indirect unit of measurement rather than a direct measurement.

Yield is a measure of the linear density of a roving (a long narrow bundle) of identical fibres. Yield is actually the inverse of linear density and is expressed in yards per pound, as it was originally used in areas that used imperial measures rather than metric measurements. There is thus an indirect relationship between tex (or denier) measurements and yield. For instance, a 735-tex fibre has a yield of 675 yards per pound, whereas a 1,100-tex fibre has a smaller yield of 450 yards per pound.

Cotton count is another way of measuring linear density. It contrasts with yield, as it is a count of the number of hanks (a hank is 7 leas, 840 yards or 770 metres) of skein material made from a particular fibre that weighs 1 pound (0.45 kilogram). The abbreviation for cotton count is Ne. By contrast, yarn length is the yarn length in metres. To calculate yarn length, multiply the cotton count by the yarn weight in kilograms and then multiply by 1,693.

If you want to convert denier to cotton count, the equation is $5315/\rho/den$, where ρ/den is the denier measurement. If you want to convert tex to cotton count, the equation is $590.5/\rho/tex$, where ρ/tex is the tex measurement. There are some other standard measurements that are used in fibre production. For instance, a thread is a length of 54 inches, a bundle is usually a measure of 10 pounds and a lea is usually a length of 80 threads. Mommes are a traditional measure of silk density. A momme is defined as the weight in pounds (or units of 0.45 kilogram) of a piece of fabric that is 45 inches wide and 100 yards long (approximately 108 square metres of fabric). One ounce per square yard is the equivalent of 35 grams per square metre or 8 mommes. The 45-inch width is used because that is a standard width used in silk production, though it can sometimes be produced in other widths, such as 55 inch, 65 inch or even 75 inch.

Habutai silk tends to be measured between 6 and 16 mommes. Standard chiffon is about 5 to 8 mommes, although chiffon made at twice the thickness will have a measurement in mommes of about 10 to 16. Crêpe de chine is about 11 to 16 mommes, gauze about 3 to 5 mommes, raw silk about 35 to 42 mommes, organza about 5 mommes and charmeuse about 15 to 25 mommes.

Thread count is a measure of how coarse or fine a fabric is, so isn't directly a measurement of linear density. However, it is relevant to the measurement of linear density.

Global Postcodes: a Partial Almanac

Afghanistan

In Afghan four-digit postcodes, the first two digits indicate the province, while the next two digits indicate the specific district or delivery zone. Kabul has 1 and 0 as the first two digits. The second two digits of 01 to 08 refer to the central Kabul City areas of Central Post Office, Macrorayan, Shahr-e-Naw, Darul Aman, Sayed Noor Mohammad Shah Mina, Dehburi, Taimani and Khairkhana. Thereafter, the postcodes with 50 upwards for their second two digits refer to districts of Kabul City; for instance, 1050 is Chahar Asyab, 1051 is Mussahi and so on. Refer to the Afghanistan postal website for a full up-to-date list.

Albania

In Albania the postal codes also have four digits and refer to specific post office branches; the first two digits indicate the central post office in a district, while the second two digits indicate the municipal post office. The first two-digit sections range from 10 for Tirana up to 97 for Sarandë, but note that there are numerous unused two-digit combinations between 10 and 97. For instance, 11, 12, 13 and 14 are unused, while 15 indicates the district of Krugë.

Algeria

In Algeria, five-digit postal codes are used. As with Afghanistan and Albania the first two digits indicate the province, but in the case of Algeria there are three digits used for a more precise indication of the exact location. A few examples: for Agouni Gueghrane the postal code is 15465; for Fougaret ez Zouia the code is 11220; for Inoughissene the code is 05240; and for Mezaourou Sidi Brahim the code is 13421. For a full list of codes refer to the Algerian post office.

Andorra

In Andorra the postal service is provided by the postal services of Spain and France. Five-digit postal codes are used, which keeps the postal codes consistent with the format used in both France and Spain, but with AD as the first two digits indicating Andorra. The full list of parishes is AD100 for Canillo, AD200 for Encamp, AD300 for Ordino, AD400 for La Massana, AD500 for Andorra la Vella, AD600 for Sant Julià de Lòria and AD700 for Escaldes-Engordany.

Argentina

Since 1998 Argentina has used the CPA (which stands for Código Postal Argentino, or Argentine Postal Code). It is a more complex system than the ones we have considered above. The first single letter indicates which of the 23 provinces of the country the address is in. For instance, Q indicates Neuquén. The next four digits indicate the city. The first of these digits indicates a general area. For instance, a CPA with 3 in this position indicates the general area of Chaco, Corrientes, Entre Ríos, Formosa, Misiones and Santa Fe. Then particular second digits indicate narrower areas, such as P31XX for Paraná or W3400 for Corrientes. Finally, the last three digits of the CPA indicate the specific block of a city or village street in which an address is located. As an example, the British Embassy in Buenos Aires has a CPA of C1425EOF.

Armenia

Armenia used to have a six-digit postal code system. In 2006 they switched to a revised four-digit system. Unlike some postal code systems that avoid using an initial zero, the Armenian system does include postal codes that start with a zero. For instance, the postal code for Berqarat is 0404. A few other examples are 1120 for Arevashat; 1415 for Verin Getashen and 2225 for Mayakovski.

A Brief Explanation of Test Match Cricket

Cricket is a game that can be played in a variety of formats, ranging from a version that lasts a few hours, up to the longest form of the game, test match cricket, which lasts for up to five days, with each day's play lasting about six or seven hours – during which players break for lunch and for tea and then continue playing.

The game is played on a large flat grass field. In the middle of the field is the pitch, a square area of carefully tended grass that is harder and flatter than the rest of the ground. At each end of the pitch there is a set of three wickets and two bails, with a popping crease marked in front of it. When the players start the game the fielding side take up positions around the field with names such as long on, midwicket, square leg, short leg, mid-off, third man and so on. There is also a wicketkeeper standing behind one set of wickets and a bowler at the opposite end (which in the first instance is called the bowler's end, although this will change after every over). For the batting team there is one batsman facing (who will face the ball when it is bowled) and one batsman at the bowler's end. The batsman is called a batsman because he or she has a bat with which he or she will attempt to hit the ball.

The bowler runs up to one end of the pitch and bowls the ball at the wickets at the other end, being careful not to overstep the popping crease because if he or she does it will be a no-ball and he or she will have to bowl the ball again. The batsman attempts to hit the ball, or at least to prevent the ball from hitting his or her wicket. If he or she hits it, or if the wicketkeeper doesn't keep the ball, the batsmen may run from one wicket to the other, in which case they score a run. The batsman may be out by being run out, caught, bowled (when the ball hits the wickets), stumped (when the wicketkeeper breaks the wicket with the ball while the batsman is out of the crease), hit wicket or leg before wicket. If he or she is out he or she leaves the field and another batsman is in. If the ball reaches the edge of the field, the batsman scores four runs, and if it reaches the edge without bouncing, he or she scores six runs. The result of each ball is recorded by the scorer. For instance, a dot ball is recorded using a dot, a single run is recorded by writing a '1', a four by writing a '4' and so on.

After the bowler has bowled the ball and the batsman has either hit it or not hit it and either been out or not out, the fielders retrieve the ball and that is the end of the ball. Now that the ball is over, the ball is dead until the bowler bowls the next ball. No one can be out when the ball is dead. The bowler should bowl six balls in an over, although if there are any no-balls he or she will bowl another ball to replace the no-ball. The batsman can't be out off a no-ball unless he or she is run out or stumped. The bowler also bowls extra balls for any wides, but not for byes (when the batsman scores without hitting the ball) or leg-byes (where the batsman scores after the ball has hit his or her leg, rather than his or her bat).

Once the bowler has bowled his or her over, play switches ends and a new bowler will bowl the next ball from the other end. The batsman who is at the bowler's end at the end of an over will face the first ball of the next over. If a batsman is caught out, then the position of the batsmen depends on where they were when the ball was caught. If the batsmen crossed, they take up a position as though a run has been scored (although a run hasn't been scored). If they haven't crossed, then the batsman at the bowler's end returns to the bowler's end (which will stop being the bowler's end if it is the end of an over).

The new bowler bowls six balls in his or her over, unless there are any no-balls or wides. Then play switches back to the other end again, and the next over may be bowled by the bowler of the first over, or by another bowler, and play continues.

A Detailed Textual Analysis
of *Don Quixote*[1]

In chapter 1, which has the title 'Which Treats of the Character and Pursuits of the Famous Gentleman Don Quixote of La Mancha', the first word is 'In'. As a preposition, this words sets the reader up to expect to be told about a situation in which something is enclosed by, surrounded by or located in something else, meaning that we need to read on to find out what this thing is. The second word is 'a', which is a form of the indefinite article in the English language, meaning that we are about to be told about something that is one example of a set of similar things. The third word is 'village', which conveys considerably more information than the previous two words and clarifies them considerably. Unless this sentence is going to take some unexpected turns we can assume that the village is the thing that something is 'in' and that we are talking only about 'a village' not 'the village'.

So within just three words we have gone from considerable uncertainty as to the direction this sentence is taking, to a sudden moment of clarity, in which we find that the first location we are being asked to think about is a village. But we still need more information to move this sentence forwards. The fourth word is 'of', which is the second preposition of the sentence. This preposition tells us that we are going to be given some information that further identifies the village because the only likely way the sentence can progress from here is to identify a place or class or quality that is possessed by the village that has been previously mentioned. We can deal with the fifth and sixth words of the sentence simultaneously, since together they form a proper name: 'La' and 'Mancha'. Depending on which edition of the book we are reading, and whether or not we paid attention to the title of the

1 This textual analysis is based on the 1885 John Ormsby translation into English.

chapter, we may already know that the person we are expecting to be the hero or protagonist of this book, Don Quixote, is from La Mancha. Alternatively, we may not know what or where La Mancha is, but if we don't, we are likely to have a strong suspicion that it is a place or region in which there are several villages, given that this village is merely 'a village' in La Mancha rather than 'the village in La Mancha'.

After the sixth word of the sentence we reach our first comma, which is a punctuation symbol that allows us a brief moment to pause and review the information we have received so far. Our expectation at this stage is that we are about to be told more about the village, or perhaps about something that happened in the village. However, the writer of this book is not shaping up to be the most direct of writers, as has already been suggested by their use of the indefinite article, so it is interesting to note that the next move is somewhat less predictable than we might expect. The seventh word, which follows the first comma, is 'the', which on its own gives us little additional information. It does, however, mark a departure from the previous use of the indefinite article and suggests we may be about to get some concrete information. The eighth word is 'name', indicating that the definite article has been used to modify this noun, which refers to the word or set of words by which a person or thing is known or can be known. This brings in the concept of reference, and the way in which things and words are connected via the naming convention and the difficulty of being truly precise about what a name refers to, whether it refers to just one person or thing, a range of persons or things, a specific thing or a class of things.

The ninth word is 'of'. This is Cervantes's first repetition of a word, and once again it is a preposition, meaning that one in every three of the words used up to this stage is a preposition. Since prepositions relate to nouns or pronouns and express a connection between other words in a clause or sentence, we may at this point conclude that the structure of the sentence is almost as important to Cervantes as the actual information.

Global Postcodes: More of Them

Australia

Australian postcodes have four digits (and it is customary to also use an abbreviation of the state or territory, such as NSW for New South Wales, in the address). As a general rule, the first two digits indicate the state or territory. For instance, the codes from 1000 to 2999 indicate addresses in New South Wales, with the exceptions of the codes from 2600 to 2619, which indicate the Australian Capital Territory, and the codes from 2900 to 2920, which also refer to the Australian Capital Territory. It is important to understand that the appropriate post office for an address, and thus the first two digits of a postcode, may sometimes be across the state or territory border from the actual address. For instance, for Alpurrurulam in the Northern Territory you would use the postcode 4825. Postcodes from 4000 to 4999 and from 9000 to 9999 generally indicate an address in Queensland, so this appears to be a Queensland postcode, but the actual delivery address would be in the Northern Territory. Another example of this kind of anomaly is 0872, the postcode that you would use for Ngaanyatjarra-Giles in Western Australia. Postcodes from 0800 to 0999 generally indicate an address in the Northern Territory, but the 0872 postcode is used for Ngaanyatjarra-Giles.

Austria

The general rule in the four-digit Austrian postal code is that the first digit indicates the region and that this generally coincides with one of the nine regions (which are called *Bundesländer*) of Austria. A postal code starting with a 1 generally refers to Vienna, 2 to Lower Austria (eastern part), 3 to Lower Austria (western part), 4 to Upper Austria, 5 to Salzburg and east Upper Austria, 6 to Tyrol and Vorarlberg but not East Tyrol, 7 to Burgenland, 8 to Styria and 9 to Carinthia and East Tyrol. The second number refers to the region of the state, the third to the route used to reach the region and the fourth to a particular post office. However, as so often happens with postal codes, there are some exceptions to the rules. For instance, the second two digits in Vienna show the district (for instance, 111X would be the eleventh district), but there is a special code for some specific locations, such as the airport (1300), and some cities close to the German border have a German postal code as well as an Austrian postal code. For a full list of postal codes, refer to the Austrian postal company, which is called Austrian Post.

Azerbaijan
Like Armenia (see p. 151) Azerbaijan used to use a six-digit postal code system but has switched to a four-digit postal code system. The first two digits indicate the administrative region, such as Neftchala District, Khojavend District or Dashkasan. Bear in mind that in administrative terms, Azerbaijan consists of 59 districts, 11 cities and the Nakhchivan Autonomous Republic. As an example of a postcode in Azerbaijan, the British embassy has a postcode of AZ1010 (where AZ simply indicates the country and the first 10 indicates Baku.

Bahrain
In Bahrain the postal codes range from 101 to 1216. However, not every three-digit number or four-digit number between 101 and 1216 is valid as a postal code. The first digit in a three-digit code and the first two digits in a four-digit code refer to one of the country's 12 municipalities, which, in this case, serve as administrative districts of the postal service. The Arabic name for the postal code in Bahrain translates more accurately as 'block number'.

Battle Tactics in the
Napoleonic Era

The era of Napoleon saw some highly significant developments in battle tactics and strategies. Napoleon had two favourite strategies: the strategy of indirect approach and the strategy of the central position. The strategy of indirect approach focused on attempts to approach the enemy in an indirect manner, while the strategy of the central position involved taking a position at the centre of the location. The strategy of indirect approach often involved using a curtain of manoeuvre. This was a strategy that involved concealing the method and direction of a manoeuvre. He used this strategy in battles at Ulm in 1805, Jena in 1806 and Friedland in 1807.

By contrast, the strategy of the central position can be described as a strategy of inferiority, which is a strategy you use in a position of relative inferiority. Napoleon sometimes used the strategy of indirect approach and the strategy of the central position interchangeably. This interchangeability was a feature of battles in 1813 at Bautzen and Lützen, though the resulting strategy was not entirely successful in these cases. The aim in such battles was to have not just a victory but a decisive victory. In responding to Napoleon's tactics of the strategy of indirect approach and the strategy of the central position, the Allies tended to rely on the concentric advance. This was an advance that had a concentric aspect to its methodology. In general, we can divide specific battle plans into two main categories: the battle of manoeuvre and the battle of attrition. The battle of manoeuvre is a tactic in which one attempts to use manoeuvres to gain an advantage, while the battle of attrition is a more attritional approach. Napoleon often relied on the battle of manoeuvre but sometimes used the battle of attrition instead.

The Jena campaign of 1806 provides us with some relevant examples of Napoleon's strategies. It lasted one month, from

6 October to 6 November. One of Napoleon's specific tactics in this campaign was the *bataillon carré* (the battalion square), which involved arraying a specific battalion in a square shape. This square could advance behind a cavalry screen in order to perform a *manoeuvre sur les derries*. Starting from the Rhine River and the Upper Danube, Napoleon's troops unexpectedly advanced to the north, with considerable success. This took the troops past the Thuringian Forest Mountains, which might have seem strategically unwise. However, given the location of the Prussian and Russian troops and supply lines, it was a well-executed strategy. There was heavy fighting at Jena and also at Auerstädt, in which the French troops mostly prevailed.

When enemy contact was encountered in these battles, the advanced guard would take up an advanced position. The light infantry would carry out infantry manoeuvres in support of the advance guard. Once the enemy army was engaged, fighting would ensue, either of the battle of manoeuvre variety or, less frequently, of the battle of attrition model. Napoleon generally chose an offensive battle formation, in which one's troops attempt to aggressively attack the opposing forces, over a defensive formation, in which one attempts to defend one's flank, centre and supply lines. However, he did sometimes choose to use defensive strategies in situations where he felt a defensive approach was more likely to be successful than an offensive approach.

Napoleon once said, 'Strategy is the art of making use of time and space'. He was less concerned about the latter than the former, although he did sometimes prioritise the latter over the former. He preferred strategies that didn't require any elements of encampment or entrenchment, preferring active strategies to inactive ones, although on a few occasions he did choose to use an inactive strategy in which his troop encamped or entrenched themselves into specific positions.

Cardboard Box Manufacturing

Etymologically speaking, cardboard is a problematic word – there is actually no single thing called cardboard. Instead, it is a portfolio concept, used to describe a set of similar materials that create a relatively solid board from a base of paper. Putting that detail to one side, how exactly are cardboard boxes manufactured?

The first thing to understand is that a cardboard box is made up of a flute, a padding layer usually made of recycled paper, which is placed between two liners made of card that may also be made from recycled paper, although the liners can sometimes be made from kraft, which is a kind of paper made from chemical pulp that is produced using the kraft process. In particular, the external liner is more likely to be made of kraft paper while the internal liner may be recycled. The liner on top of the fluting forms the typical corrugated-board effect, due to the corrugation of the fluting distorting the surface. For a smoother finish, kraft paper made from softwood trees with long fibres is used. Long fibres have a better resistance to tearing or bursting.

Kraft paper can have a variety of appearances, depending on the tree it comes from. Some types of kraft paper are more beige, some are a slight darker brown and some are a slightly more yellowish shade of brown. The internal liners are often made of test paper from hardwood trees, which have shorter fibres – on their own these would be relatively weak and abrasive, but because the outer liner provides greater resistance to tears and bursts, the use of a weaker paper internally is not problematic. The fluted paper that forms the layer between the inner and outer layer can be made from either test paper or kraft paper, each of which would create a slightly different texture of board.

To understand the variation in types of paper, it is important to understand the paper-making process. This starts with the production of wood, which comes from trees (preferably from trees that have been sustainably produced). The wood is cut, milled, lumbered, debarked and transported, and then turned into chips. The chips are then put through a process of either mechanical pulping or chemical pulping. Mechanical pulping is a method of pulping using a machine that grinds the chips into pulp. Chemical pulping involves using chemicals to chemically reduce the chips into pulp. The chemicals used are either sulphates or sulphites. Sulphate pulping is a more common process – an alkaline solution is used to create a stronger variety of pulp.

The kraft paper is then produced from the pulp – it will usually be one of a variety of shades of brown but it can also be bleached using a chemical bleach to produce kraft that is white, off-white or grey. Different shades of grey can be achieved, depending on the shade of brown one starts with, which, in turn, depends on the type of tree that was used to produce the wood chips.

On the other hand, if recycled paper is being used, then the process starts with any one of a variety of types of recycled waste. For instance, one might use chip liners, which are made from recycled fibre (these are quite weak, so are mostly used in fluting). Alternatively, semi-recycled paper can be made from a mixture of recycled waste and wood chips.

When it comes to the fluting that is going to end up in between the external and internal liner papers, rolls of paper are fed through a corrugated roller machine, in order to add corrugation to the paper. There are several types of fluting board – you can use B flute or R flute, which can also be referred to as S board or M board. In several important aspects, including print quality and emission measurements, R flute is a 30 per cent improvement on B flute. You may also see boxes that are labelled as having AB flute or BC flute. This labelling is used to distinguish double-layered cardboard boxes from single-layered cardboard boxes. The final stage of the process is to apply adhesive to the fluting and the liners so that they adhere to one another and to complete the process of making the box.

Metric and Imperial Measurements of Screws

Screws come in a variety of types. It is important to use the right screw for a particular job; otherwise, it may be hard to screw or unscrew the screw. Depending on the job you are undertaking, you may want to use a wood screw, single or twin thread screws, twin fine thread screws, passivated screws, zinc and passivated yellow screws, a brass crosshead, a brass crosshead countersunk screw, drywall screws, stainless steel self-tappers or zinc-plated self-tappers, concrete and masonry self-tapping screws, zinc or brass roundhead screws, chipboard countersunk screws, brass or black Japanned screws, zinc-plated twin thread roofing screws or decking screws.

Some standard abbreviations for screws include:

ST: self-tapping – screws that do not require a hole
TT: twin thread – a screw with two threads instead of one
TFT: twin fine thread – a screw with two fine threads
ZP: zinc plating – a screw plated with zinc for extra protection from the possibility of corrosion
ZYPL: zinc and yellow passivated – a screw with a layer of zinc plating and a layer of yellow passsivated plating

The main difference between metric and imperial sizes for screws is that metric screw sizes give a diameter and length in millimetres, while imperial screw sizes are based on a gauge size and length in inches.

A 3mm diameter in metric is equivalent to an imperial gauge size 4. This size is generally available in sizes of 12mm (½ in), 16mm (⅝ in), 20mm (¾ in), 25mm (1 in), 30mm (1¼ in) and 40mm (1½ in).

A 3.5mm in metric is equivalent to an imperial gauge size 6. This size is generally available in sizes of 12mm (½ in), 16mm (⅔ in), 20mm (¾ in), 25mm (1 in), 30mm (1¼ in) and 40mm (1½ in).

A 4mm metric size is equivalent to an imperial gauge size 8. This size is generally available in sizes of 12mm (½ in), 16mm (⅝ in), 20mm (¾ in), 25mm (1 in), 30mm (1¼ in), 40mm (1½ in), 45mm (1¾ in), 50mm (2 in), 60mm (2½ in) and 70mm (2¾ in).

A 4.5mm metric size is equivalent to an imperial gauge size 9. This size is generally available in sizes of 25mm (1 in), 30mm (1¼ in), 40mm (1½ in), 45mm (1¾ in), 50mm (2 in), 60mm (2½ in), 70mm (2¾ in) and 75mm (3 in).

A 5mm metric size is equivalent to an imperial gauge size 10. This size is generally available in sizes of 25mm (1 in), 30mm (1¼ in), 40mm (1½ in), 45mm (1¾ in), 50mm (2 in), 60mm (2½ in), 70mm (2¾ in), 75mm (3 in), 80mm (3¼ in), 90mm (3½ in) and 100mm (4 in).

A 6mm metric size is equivalent to an imperial gauge size 12. This size is generally available in sizes of 30mm (1¼ in), 40mm (1½ in), 45mm (1¾ in), 50mm (2 in), 60mm (2½ in), 70mm (2¾ in), 75mm (3 in), 80mm (3¼ in), 90mm (3½ in), 100mm (4 in), 110mm (4⅝ in), 130mm (5⅓ in) and 150mm (6 in).

Above a 6mm size, most manufacturers don't continue to provide screws with sizes that rise in increments of ½mm or 1mm. The most commonly produced sizes are 10mm, 12mm, 16mm, 20mm, 25mm, 30mm, 35mm, 40mm, 45mm, 50mm, 60mm, 50mm, 80mm, 90mm and so on.

Critique of Pure Reason by
Immanuel Kant: a Brief Summary

Critique of Pure Reason starts with Kant's approach to aesthetics, a term that he uses with an approximate meaning that differs from the usual meaning of the term. For Kant, the aesthetic can be subdivided into intuitive and conceptual aspects, meaning that we have to distinguish between intuitive perceptions and conceptualised perceptions. He uses the German word *Anschauung* to refer to 'intuition' – it suggests that the term 'intuition' is being used in a sense closer to the English word 'perception'.

Kant's intention is to understand the human mind as an active participant in intuition and conceptualisation, rather than as a passive recipient of perceptions. As well as *Anschauung* it is important to be aware that Kant uses the German word *Verstand* to describe the interaction of reason and conceptualisation. He goes on to analyse the various kinds of knowledge that we might be able to derive from our perceptions and intuition, or from our *Anschauung* and *Verstand*. A statement (and reference to facts containing a subject and an object) can be regarded, for instance, as analytic if it is tautologous or can be analysed in such a way as to show that the predicate is contained by the subject. If a statement isn't analytic, then, for Kant, it must by definition be synthetic. It is also important to distinguish between statements that are *a priori* and *a posteriori*, which is a distinction between whether their truth is testable or determined by experience or not. Generally, analytic statements are *a priori*, while all *a posteriori* statements are synthetic, as their subject doesn't contain their predicate.

However, the crucial question that immediately strikes most readers of Kant is whether or not it is possible for a statement to be both synthetic and *a priori*. Kant's claim is ultimately going to be that the most crucial statements that it is possible to make using philosophical language will indeed be synthetic at the same time as being *a priori* (in other words, neither analytic nor *a posteriori*). He points out, for instance, that when Hume denies that synthetic *a priori* statements are possible, this is, ironically, a synthetic *a priori* statement in itself! Similar arguments could be applied to many statements that would later be made by the logical positivists.

The next key distinction Kant makes is that between phenomena and noumena. The phenomenal is the real world as we understand it from our perceptions and intuition, or from our *Anschauung* and *Verstand*. The entire notion of objectivity is, of course, ground in our perception and intuitions of phenomena. The noumenal is the world as it is regardless of our perceptions, intuition, *Anschauung* or *Verstand* of how it is. In other words, the noumenal world simply is. The obvious consequence is that the world we know is the phenomenal world, which is related to the noumenal world but is not in and of itself the noumenal world, which means that we cannot directly perceive the noumenal world.

This important distinction will be revisited when we start to understand Kant's theory of transcendental knowledge. The transcendental deduction is one that is beyond experience. For instance, the deduction from phenomenal to noumenal or subjective to objective might be considered to be transcendent. Transcendental could be defined as being an intuition concerning our specific mode of cognition, thus, like other words such as 'aesthetic', 'objective' and 'reason', Kant is using a word in a non-standard meaning, which means that we must always remember to forget our usual perception of the meaning of the words while we are reading *Critique of Pure Reason*. A similar distinction applies when we come to the distinction between 'pure' and 'empirical'. For Kant, a concept is pure if it is not empirical and thus if it is transcendental and abstractly arrived at from experience.

Some Recent Developments
in String Theory

- In 1984 K. Kikkawa and M. Yamasaki of Osaka University demonstrated that if you 'curl up' one of the extra dimensions into a circle with radius R, the applicable theory is the same as if we curl up this dimension with radius 1/R.

- If we apply this T-duality to various superstrings, we reduce five types of string theory down to three types.

- In the 1990s Juan Maldacena showed that string theory that included gravity in five dimensions could be seen as being equivalent to a four-dimensional quantum field theory in four dimensions.

- The consequent 'AdS/CFT' could provide a superior way to deal with gravity by connecting it to quantum field theory.

- However, in 1995 Edward Witten showed that the string theories known as type I, type IIA and type IIB, and the two heterotic string theories, SO(32) and $E_8 \times E_8$), could be reduced to a single theory, M-theory.

- In nine dimensions type IIA and IIB strings are identical, and so are $E_8 \times E_8$ and SO(32) strings.

- S-duality and U-duality have helped define the duality between the perturbative and non-perturbative parts of string theory.

- In 1998 Alain Connes, Michael R. Douglas and Albert Schwarz made some significant contributions to the relation between matrix models and M-theory by using a non-commutative quantum field theory.

- Edward Witten (with Paul Townsend) has also demonstrated a duality between ten-dimensional type IIA strings and 11-dimensional supergravity.

- Cumrun Vafa and Andrew Strominger have shown that the Bekenstein–Hawking entropy of a black hole is accounted for by solitonic states of superstring theory.

- Vafa is also partially responsible for the Gopakumar–Vafa conjecture, which suggests that the Gromov–Witten invariants of a Calabi–Yau 3-fold can be canonically expressed in terms of integer invariants (which we can call BPS numbers).

The Varying Sizes and Colours of Bricks in Great Britain

- Bricks generally need to be small enough to be held in one hand while the mortar is applied with the other hand. A small brick size will mean a longer bricklaying process, as more bricks will be needed for a particular area.

- Brick-making in eastern England dates back to the late thirteenth and early fourteenth centuries. Bricks during this period were relatively small, but some early medieval bricks were as big as 13 in × 6 in × 2 in.

- Most fifteenth-century bricks were about 9½ in × 4½ in × 2 in, and a charter in 1571 specified the closely related size of 9 in × 4½ in × 2¼ in.

- In the late seventeenth and early eighteenth centuries, the process of brick manufacture was improved, as blended clay and better moulding led to bricks of a more consistent size.

- In the late seventeenth century, common colours for bricks were red, purple and grey. By 1730 brownish and pinkish grey bricks were also common. Bricks during this period were still smaller and less consistent in size than modern bricks.

- In the mid-eighteenth century, most bricks were grey, although yellow marl London bricks came into fashion in about 1800.

- From the mid-eighteenth century onwards, mechanised manufacturing meant deeper clays were used for being pressed into dense and larger brick sizes.

- In the eighteenth century, Parliament once mandated a brick size 8½ in × 4 in × 2½ in, which is equivalent to the modern metric (see below).

- The government introduced a brick tax in 1784. It was paid per brick, so brick-makers started making much larger bricks.

- Joseph Wilkes of Measham went to an extreme, producing bricks double the normal size (approximately 110mm × 110mm × 235mm or 4⅜ in × 4⅜ in × 9¼ in). They were nicknamed Jumbies or Wilkes's Gobbs.

- In response, the government set an upper limit of 150 cubic inches (10 in × 5 in × 3 in) for a brick, but bricks of the period remained larger than earlier bricks had been.

The Mechanics of Bowling Alleys

Early bowling alleys had the pins reset by hand, which is a complex and labour-intensive process. The first automatic pinsetter was patented by Gottfried Schmidt, and manufactured by the American Machine and Foundry Company (AMF) in 1946. It weighed nearly 2 tons and was 9 feet (2.7 metres) tall.

In the ensuing decades automatic pinsetters have become increasingly lightweight and efficient. A pinsetter consists of four main parts: the sweep, the pin elevator, the pin distributor and the pin table. The original set of ten pins are collectively known as a rack, and each game is made up of ten frames, in which you have two balls. The pinsetter is designed to reset the rack at the start of each frame, and to clear away any pins that have been knocked over.

There are 4,000 individual components in an automatic pinsetter. The most up-to-date pinsetters use a small scanner camera that is mounted over the lane. Another type takes data from the scanner and runs it through an algorithm in order to establish which pins have been knocked down. The system passes this information to the pinsetter.

In earlier pinsetters, such scanners weren't available, so the pinsetting mechanism came with a modification that employed mechanical fingers to determine which pins had been knocked down. This was a delicate task as it needed to be performed without knocking down the surviving pins.

If any pins remain standing after the first ball, the pinsetter is designed to pick up the remaining pins and clear away the pins that have been knocked down but that haven't fallen into the gutter, and then replace the remaining pins back on the lane correctly.

A sensor located in front of the pins triggers the activity of the pinsetter, following a tiny delay to allow the ball to strike the pins or the back of the lane if it has missed the pins and landed in the ball pit. The ball pit is the area directly behind the rack of pins that receives the ball and any pins that have been swept off the lane after the impact of the ball.

First, the sweep: a rectangular sheet of metal that comes down in front of the pins to protect the pinsetter from being hit by any balls that are incorrectly thrown before the pins have been reset. Now that the sweep is in place, the pinsetter moves down to pick up the remaining pins. The pin table, a part of the pinsetter that has ten holes, is lowered on top of the pins. The ten holes are designed to fit snugly over the remaining pins and to secure them while the loose pins are cleared away. The pin table grips the pins and picks them up in the spotting tongs.

At this stage, the pinsetter automatically ascertains how many pins have been picked up and sends this information to the automatic scoring software. Now that the pinsetter is safely raised, the sweep is moved to the back of the lane in such a way that any loose pins will be swept into the ball pit. These pins are swept from the ball pit into the pin elevator, which elevates the pins into a position from which they can be reset by the pinsetter.

The sweep returns to the guard position to once again protect the pinsetter from any incorrectly thrown balls. Now the pin table is lowered and the spotting tongs loosen, allowing the pins to gently fall back into their original positions. The pinsetter then rises back to its original position, leaving the correct array of remaining positions. Now the sweep is raised once more and the pins are available for the next ball. At this stage, pins that have been elevated in the pin elevator are manoeuvred precisely into position to fill the pin table with ten pins ready for the next player.

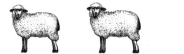

How Many Are There Now?

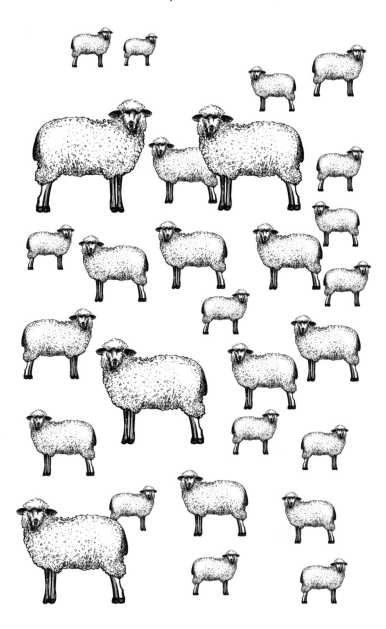

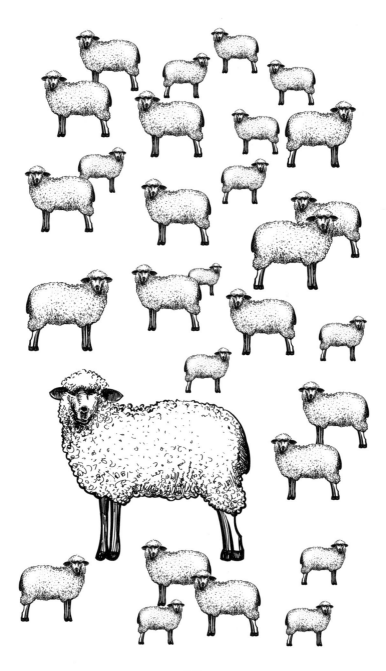

Breakfast in the Ancient World

Archaeological evidence suggests that Stone Age humans ate grains for breakfast over 20,000 years ago. They also ate wild grains as a significant part of their everyday diet. The wheat and barley they ate was quite similar to the wheat and barley we eat today. A large grinding stone found by archaeologists, which looked like a big mortar and pestle, suggests that the cereals were ground before being prepared. As well as cereal, Stone Age people ate leaves and drank water. A typical day's breakfast might consist of cereal, leaves and a selection of nuts and berries.

By the Bronze Age humans were using honey in their cooking, especially for breakfast. Crop seeds were ground into flour to make bread. A variety of nuts and seeds would be added. They also drank water and other drinks with their breakfast.

By the time of the ancient Greeks the typical diet in the region consisted of foods that were readily available in that region. The typical breakfast, eaten after sunrise, was made up of bread and possibly cakes. Honey was their main sweetener. Some Greeks would add olives, cheese, figs or dried fish. The wine that was drunk with breakfast was watered down. Many people had access to fish, which was occasionally eaten for breakfast. There wasn't a strong culture of animal husbandry, so meat was only available at certain times of the year in particular situations. The ancient Greeks mostly ate with their fingers rather than with eating utensils.

Breakfast habits among the Romans were not hugely different to the breakfast habits of the Greeks, although they depended more on the crops from their own region. At dawn breakfast was prepared by the cooks. Breakfast was known as the *ientaculum*. Wealthy Romans might eat bread, honey and fruit, which could be accompanied by a glass of wine or perhaps plain water. They also ate cheese, olives and raisins for breakfast. However, for most ordinary Romans, breakfast would have been just plain water and a piece of bread.

Ancient Aztec and Mayan civilisations ate chocolate as well as various nuts, grains and fruits. They primarily used chocolate after the harvest of the cacao beans, brewing it into a hot drink. Over time it became a breakfast staple, eaten alongside grains and nuts.

In another part of the world, in China, rice was the first grain that was extensively farmed. There is evidence of rice farming in China from about 5000 BC. Just as today, it was prepared by being boiled in water until it was soft enough to eat. Rice wine has been also been made in China over the centuries and may also have been a significant breakfast ingredient. By 4500 BC people in China were also farming millet and boiling it into a kind of porridge. By about 3500 BC tea was being cultivated, and it wasn't long before tea was the standard breakfast drink in China. To their breakfast rice, the ancient Chinese added fruit, nuts or vegetables of various varieties.

Early Indians ate a variety of foods that were common in their region. Fruits, grains, wild berries, meat and fish were the most common foods available for breakfast consumption. As agriculture developed they also started to consume farmed crops and pulses. The most fertile regions of ancient India were in the river valleys. Like the Chinese, rice was a staple food and would be eaten at various meals with cooked lentils and vegetables. The early Indus Valley Civilisation is recorded as breakfasting on wheat and rice and lentils. Some meat would also have been consumed, but this changed by around 300 BC, when many became vegetarians. The vegetarian breakfast favoured at this stage was mainly wheat flatbreads or a kind of flatbread made of chickpeas, yoghurt and vegetables. As a drink to accompany this food they preferred to drink plain water.

The Motion of Sand Dunes

The clearest technical definition of sand is that it is an aggregate of rock fragments. If we need to discuss different types of sand, there are a few ways of grading its size. The International Organization for Standardization (ISO) simply grades sand as fine (0.063mm to 0.2mm), medium (0.2mm to 0.63mm) and coarse (0.63mm to 2.0mm). For a more precise grading system, we can use the Krumbein phi scale[1], which is commonly used in the USA. The five subcategories are: very fine sand (0.0625mm to 0.125mm in diameter); fine sand (0.125mm to 0.25m); medium sand (0.25mm to 0.5mm); coarse sand (0.5mm to 1mm); and very coarse sand (1mm to 2mm).

Sand originally comes from fragmented rock and is an intermediate phase between pebbles and clay. In inland settings and coastal settings that aren't tropical the most common element is silica (silicon dioxide, or SiO_2), which can be in the form of quartz or in other forms. A dune is just the name for a hill of loose sand. Dunes can be formed by the wind (which is known as formation by aeolian processes) or water (which is known as formation by fluvial processes). Dunes also form on the beds of rivers, lakes and oceans. Dunes tend to be longer on the windward side, as the sand on this side tends to be pushed up the dune, leaving the dune with a significantly shorter side in the lee of the wind.

The valley or trough between two sand dunes is called a slack. Where an area contains numerous sand dunes it is called a dune field. There is a wide variety of dune shapes. Crescent or transverse dunes (also called barchans) are formed where the wind blows in a consistent manner from the same direction. A crescent dune moves and reshapes faster than other types of dune

[1] This scale defines size using the equation $\Phi = -\log_2 D$ where D is the particle size in millimetres. On this scale, value of Φ for sand varies from -1 to $+4$, and the subcategories start and finish at the whole number divisions.

because the movement is consistently in the same direction. Sand is blown from the top of the dune and falls down the far side of the dune, then the process continues until the dune gradually shifts in position.

A group of crescent dunes was observed in the 1950s in China in the Ningxia Province that showed that the dunes were moving by about 100 metres per year. Experiments in the Western Desert in Egypt have reached a similar conclusion. There are barchan dunes on Mars, which are the result of a constant wind direction on the surface of the planet.

A different type of dune is a linear dune, which is a linear shape, of up to 150 kilometres in width. A star dune is a pyramidal shape with faces down with sand slips on three arms or more. These faces radiate out from the centre of the dune, forming a kind of pyramidal shape, thus the name. Pyramidal dunes are more common when the wind is not consistently in the same direction.

Oval or circular mounds don't have the kinds of faces that are characteristic of star dunes. Dome dunes are dunes that are dome-shaped – this is a relatively unusual shape for a dune to be. Parabolic dunes are mounds of sand with parabolic shapes. They are formed when the particular local situation leads to the formation of a U-shaped depression. Compound parabolic dunes are similar to parabolic dunes, but they have sets of trailing arms that distinguish them from a normal parabolic dune. They tend to form at 90 degrees to the prevailing wind. Longitudinal or seif dunes run parallel to the prevailing wind, and can be formed where a larger dune has started to collapse. They have sharp crests and can often be found in deserts with conditions similar to the Sahara.

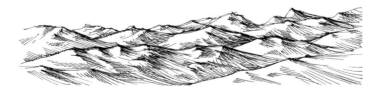

Some English Language Facts

Aegilops (8 letters long) is the longest word to have all of its letters arranged in alphabetical order. Shorter words of this kind include beefily and billowy (7 letters), abhors, accent, access, almost, biopsy, bijoux, billow, chintz, effort and ghosty (all 6 letters). Spoonfeed (at 9 letters long) is the longest word to have all of its letters in reverse alphabetical order.

Nonsupports (11 letters long) is the longest word in the English language that only uses letters from the second half of the alphabet. The 10-letter runners-up include prosupport, soupspoons and zoosporous.

Overnumerousnesses (18 letters) is the longest English word that consists of only letters that lack ascenders, descenders and dots in lower case. Overnervousnesses has 17 letters. Sixteen-letter words of this kind include curvaceousnesses and overnumerousness, while erroneousnesses, nonconcurrences, overnervousness and verrucosenesses have 15 letters each.

Dermatoglyphics, misconjugatedly and uncopyrightable are the longest English words in which no letter appears more than once (15 letters each). The 14-letter runners-up include ambidextrously, benzhydroxamic, hydromagnetics, hydropneumatic, pseudomythical, schizotrypanum, sulphogermanic, troublemakings, undiscoverably and vesiculography.

Esophagographers is the longest English word in which each of the letters occurs exactly twice (16 letters). Shorter words with the same pattern of twin letters include scintillescent (14 letters), happenchance and shanghaiings (12 letters), arraigning, concisions, intestines and horseshoer (10 letters).

In the word sestettes each of the letters occurs three times.

A simple code is to use a Caesar Cipher (see p. 116) to encode secret messages. If you use the letter 13 places further on in the alphabet to code a word ('a' becomes 'n', 'b' becomes 'o', 'c' becomes 'p' and so on), then this code is symmetrical, meaning that encryption and decoding are the same process. The longest known words that become another proper word using this system are abjurer and nowhere, which encode to one another.

Eunoia is the shortest English word that contains all five principal vowels (excluding 'y'). Longer words that achieve the same feat include adoulie, douleia, Eucosia, eulogia, eunomia, eutopia, miaoued, moineau, Sequoia and suoidea (7 letters each).

Caesious is the shortest English word containing all five principal vowels in alphabetical order. Tied for second place with 9 letters each are acheilous, acheirous, aerobious, arsenious, arterious, autecious, facetious and parecious.

Suoidea (7 letters long) is the shortest English word containing all five principal vowels in reverse alphabetical order. Following a long way behind are duoliteral and unoriental (10 letters), subcontinental (14 letters), neuroepithelial and uncomplimentary (15 letters).

Twyndyllyngs is the longest word in the English language without any of the five principal vowels (at 12 letters), making do with only 'y's. The singular twyndyllyng has 11 letters, symphysy has 8 letters, while gypsyfy, gypsyry, nymphly and rhythms have 7 letters each. Strengthlessnesses is the longest word in the English language that uses a single repeated vowel (18 letters). In second place come defenselessnesses (17 letters), pursued by strengthlessness (16 letters), defenselessness (15 letters) and degenerescence (14 letters). There are no words that achieve this feat with any other vowel that are more than 13 letters long.

Institutions of the European Union:
an Introduction

In the European Union the political structure is closely tied to the structure of the various administrative and political institutions in the system. The European Council and the Council of the European Union are two different institutions in which national administrations oversee the other institutions of the European Union, while those administrations and agencies implement and oversee policy in general.

The European Council is composed of the political leaders of member states, and the President of the European Commission is also a member. It meets every three months, but sometimes more often than that. It deals with general policy and administrative objectives. *The European Commission* deals with a combination of political and administrative tasks. It proposes new legislation, manages policy, monitors compliance and represents the EU in certain situations. The College of Commissioners has 28 members, one of whom comes from each and every member state. The Commission President is the political leader of the College of Commissioners. The Commission President is nominated by the European Council.

College members are nominated by national governments, and approved by the European Parliament. Each Commission department has a Directorate-General. The Directorate-General is in charge of the particular policy being overseen by that department of the Commission. *The Council of the European Union*, which is sometimes called the Council of Ministers, is a law-making body within the administrative structure of the European Union. National delegations make up working groups, the Committee of Permanent Representatives and subcommittees of ministers. *The European Parliament* is also a law-making body. It proposes legislative proposals, which are considered by committees of the

Parliament. *The Court of Justice of the European Union* analyses the interpretation and application of the European Union's treaties, considers the legality of EU laws, and gives advice to subcommittees and national administrations concerning the fine print of EU law. *The General Court* is another judicial institution of the European Union, which considers different aspects of legislative issues to the Court of Justice of the European Union.

Laws are passed by a combination of the European Council and the European Parliament, either of which may veto a legislative proposal. The European Commission makes policy proposals. These then go through an extensive process of being considered by committees and taken to consultations. If the European Commission promotes a policy, it is considered for consultation by the European Council and the European Parliament. At this stage the European Council and the European Parliament must both agree on every word of the legislative proposal; otherwise, the process of consultation and committee consideration will continue. There are numerous other important institutions and inter-institutional bodies that play particular administrative or legislative roles in the European Union. These include the European Central Bank, which is the central bank of the European Union. The European External Action Service deals with consultation, consistency and coordination of the external action of the European Union. The European Economic and Social Committee deals with economic and social aspects of administration. The European Committee of the Regions deals with administrative issues concerning the regions of the European Union. The European Investment Bank deals with administration that concerns the European Investment Fund and investment in general in the European Union. The European Data Protection Supervisor deals with issues of data protection. The European School of Administration deals with a variety of administration issues within the institutions of the European Union.

How to Play 'Chopsticks'

'Chopsticks' (also known as the 'Celebrated Chop Waltz') is a well-known simple piece of music for the piano written by Euphemia Allen in 1877 using the pseudonym Arthur de Lulli. It can theoretically be played with the two hands in a chopping position, with the little fingers striking the keys. There are also three-handed variations available, as composed by Alexander Borodin, César Cui, Nikolai Rimsky-Korsakov and Anatoly Lyadov in 1879. Their acquaintance Modest Petrovich Mussorgsky declined their invitation for him to do likewise, regarding it as a pointless waste of his time.

To play the piece, locate middle C on a piano, then find the F and G above middle C. Play these two notes together six times. The rhythm is a staccato waltz rhythm, so the six repetitions of the note make up two bars.

Next, move your left hand one note down to the E note and play another six notes. These six notes repeat the same rhythm as the first six notes of the piece. Again, it is a consistent waltz beat lasting across two bars.

For the following six notes, which once again repeat the staccato waltz rhythm from the first four bars, move both hands. The right hand goes up two notes to the B above middle C, while the left hand goes down one note to the D above middle C.

The next two bars are more complicated. The first bar consists of a repetition of the staccato waltz rhythm for three notes on middle C (with the left hand) and the C above middle C (with the right hand). Then for the last three notes of the double bar section of the piece (the eighth bar in total) there is a descending phrase in the right hand accompanied by an ascending phrase in the left hand. This keeps up the same rhythm as the first twenty-one notes of the piece. First you play middle C and the C above middle C (as on the previous three notes), then you play D in the left hand and B in the right hand, then you play E in the left hand and A in the right hand.

At this stage you play a reprise of the first twenty-one notes. Start on the F and G above middle C. Play these two notes together six times in the same staccato waltz rhythm that we have been using throughout the piece so far.

Next, move your left hand one note down to the E note and play another six notes in the same staccato waltz rhythm. Then move your hands to the B above middle C and the D above middle C. Then once again play three notes on middle C (with the left hand) and the C above middle C (with the right hand). You might like to slow the rhythm down very slightly on these last three notes to introduce an element of suspense. Then for the final note of this section of the piece simply play the same two notes, middle C and the C above middle C, but hold the notes down for two beats rather than continuing with the staccato waltz rhythm. Again, you may want to count this bar fairly slowly compared to the usual tempo of the piece.

The next section changes rhythm slightly. It is still a waltz, but the notes are played in groups of two, with the third of every three beats left as a pause. To make life more complicated, the first of the two notes played comes on the last beat of the previous bar. So after you have held down the middle C and C above middle C for two beats in the sixteenth bar of the piece, as previously described, you jump up to play the C above middle C and the E above the C above middle C for one note, then on the first beat of the seventeenth bar, play the D above the C above middle C and the B above middle C (and hold this note for a pause on the second beat of the seventeenth bar). Then using the same rhythm, play the A above middle C and the C above middle C for the third beat of this bar, and move down to the G and the B for two beats.

In the next bar we return to playing three notes as in earlier bars. On the last beat of the bar, repeat the G and the B, then repeat this combination and continue.

ABOUT THE AUTHORS

Professor K. McCoy specializes in the analysis of hypnotic states and somnambulism. She lives on the coast and spends one hour every day, except Mondays, moving rocks to build a sea wall.

Dr Hardwick is an expert in stereotypical lethargy. He is one of the world's foremost authorities on and curators of screwdrivers.